Health & Happiness

Dr Arien van der Merwe

Tafelberg

Also available by the same author:

To Health! 1997, *HSLM Publishers*
Geluk & Gesondheid 1999, *Tafelberg Publishers*
Choose Wellness! (CD-ROM) 2001, *Modern Publishers*
FAQ All About Series 2001, *Formule Naturelle Publishing*

Cover design Etienne van Duyker
Design Etienne van Duyker, Alinea Studio, Cape Town
Printed and bound by NBD, Drukkery Street, Cape Town, South Africa
First edition 1999
Second edition, first impression 2001

ISBN 0 624 04037 2

I suggest that the body and soul react to each other in sympathy. A change in the state of the soul would necessarily have an effect on the body and vice versa.

Aristotle

Let food be your medicine.

Hippocrates

First: Do no harm!

Hippocrates

Health is our greatest gift and our most precious possession.

Arien van der Merwe

Disclaimer

The information and recommendations in this book are intended to guide, inform and educate readers in the natural ways of restoring the body, mind and soul to optimal health by means of stress management, the role and functions of micronutrients, choosing the correct supplements and leading a healthy lifestyle. We are all responsible for our own health and happiness. Discuss your specific needs, symptoms and medical condition with an informed doctor or health care practitioner for your personal requirements.

For my husband Paul and my children – Léan, Anri and Stephni –
for all their love, support and patience.

Contents

Preface

My involvement in health and complementary options goes back many years. As a qualified medical doctor, I soon became frustrated and disillusioned with treating only the symptoms of disease without knowing the real reason of how and why disease develops. As I gained more practical experience, I began to realise that stress lies at the root of most chronic Western diseases. That is why the introductory chapters of this book deal with stress and how to manage it. Many diseases can be managed and alleviated by boosting the function of systems in the body with the correct micronutrients (vitamins, minerals, amino acids, essential fatty acids and medicinal herbs) to lead the body back to improved function and health. Natural healing methods are very effective in gently restoring people to health with few (or no) side effects. Many symptomatic orthodox medicines often do the body and soul more harm than good and cause side effects that have to be treated with more medication.

People who became aware of their responsibility for their own health and of certain facts surrounding the health of the body, emotions, mind and soul will also become more spiritually aware. This helps them in their search for knowledge, happiness and fulfilment. The conscious decision to take herbs or vitamins helps us to take responsibility for our own health. Like so many before me who have chosen to follow complementary medical options, I realised that the most important part of getting better is the knowledge that we can all take control of our own health. As soon as we stop being victims, we are liberated from our restrictive ideas and are able to live fullfilling lives in a state of spiritual and physical joy – this is our birthright.

There are many books available on vitamins, minerals and their role in health, but they all fail to give clarity on the exact health requirements of the average South African family.

I hope that this book takes the guesswork and uncertainty out of food supplementation. The book is organised according to the different systems of the body to show you exactly which micronutrients support that system. Quantities, ratios and how the different micronutrients work together in synergy will further assist you in determining your needs and those of others. This book is an improved, revised version of my first book, *To Health!* It contains many new chapters, such as the specific needs of pregnant and breastfeeding women, children, participation in sport and natural methods for weight management. Case studies will confirm the practical application and use of the suggestions in this book. There is also information on well-researched medicinal herbs that will offer you natural alternatives. The list of references provides further reading material.

The classification of the body into different systems is not intended to imply that we can simply divide the body into separate compartments. For practical reasons it is useful to look at specific systems because in families there is often a genetic weakness in a specific system. During stress this specific system of the body will first show loss of function and eventually become diseased. Genetically, the weak links in the enzyme chains are the first ones to break. If the system is repaired by making lifestyle adaptations, managing stress and learning from our disease processes, our chances of recovery and an improved quality of life are so much greater.

The information and recommendations in this book are intended as guidelines for using micronutrients, adopting a healthy lifestyle and managing stress – we are all responsible for own health and wellbeing. Discuss your specific symptoms and medical conditions with your doctor (who should have some knowledge about complementary medical options) to get advice and recommendations concerning your personal health problems.

Introduction

So many people in our modern society suffer from chronic diseases, that the time has come to take stock. Despite all our technological advances and research, there is little hope of curing diseases like cancer, allergies, chronic infections, cardiovascular disorders, high cholesterol, arthritis, diabetes and chronic respiratory problems.

Scientific and medical advances have enabled us to restrict childhood infectious diseases and to a large extent eliminate diseases such as smallpox. We can diagnose and treat cancer much earlier, surgical techniques and anaesthetics have been improved and most people are far more aware of vaccination and matters of hygiene.

Throughout the world orthodox conventional medical doctors save thousands of lives after motorcar accidents, difficult deliveries and foetal distress in childbirth, acute heart attacks and strokes, serious sports injuries, assaults, life-threatening infections such as meningitis and pyelonephritis (kidney infection) and acute bronchospasm (asthma attacks). Lives are saved daily because of organ transplants. In such cases the only solution is conventional Western medical care and it really can achieve amazing results.

Orthodox medicine however, can offer little relief for the chronic diseases that most of us suffer from. In the face of increased medical costs and health insurance claims, another option (complementary and co-operative) is urgently needed to restrict the side effects associated with most medicines and the increased resistance of bacteria to antibiotics, which has reached almost epidemic proportions. Even at grassroots' level people are becoming increasingly disillusioned and dissatisfied with the current situation.

A look at the complaints of people who are likely to consult the average general practice in one day tells its own story:

- Self-limiting infections: More than 90% of viral and bacterial infections are self-limiting. This means that the body can be left to heal itself. The disease will follow its natural course and in most cases balance and wellbeing will be restored.
- Psychosomatic or mind-body diseases as they are known today:

These are the diseases that originate in the mind and manifest as physical disease processes. Examples are chronic stress that leads to complaints such as eczema, ulcers and hypertension (high blood pressure).

- Chronic diseases: Arthritis, diabetes, psoriasis, asthma, bronchitis and hypertension are diseases that usually remain in a state of balance, but flare up during times of increased stress.
- Acute diseases, trauma and accidents, heart attacks, acute bronchospasm, strokes, croup, meningitis, acute appendicitis and acute bowel obstruction: In this category orthodox (Western) medicine saves lives every day. A person who suffers a serious head injury cannot waste time being treated by a medical herb – drastic measures are needed to save the person's life, for example by stopping any bleeding in the brain.

What we often do not realise is that 90-95% of all patients fall into the first three categories. All these people would benefit from a more natural approach to assist in restoring health to the affected system of the body. Medical doctors will always be needed to give advice on the seriousness of the disease, confirm or make the correct diagnosis and monitor the progress of the disease. Patients are very appreciative of doctors who are prepared and able to offer a little more than simply treating the symptoms.

Medical doctors have the necessary medical training to ensure their patients' piece of mind. They know when a patient falls into the 5-10 per cent of consultations where drastic measures are needed to save a life (the fourth category). A mistake that people in the West often make is to think that most patients fall into the last group. Most patients will recover on their own, especially if they focus on nutritional status, stress management, lifestyle control and the right natural remedies such as herbs and supplements and getting the correct advice from their health care provider.

The life situation we find ourselves in, genetic or inherited factors, education and life experiences both as children and adults can have strange consequences. Most of us have a lifestyle that makes too many demands on our body and mind. By improving our lifestyle, acquiring correct eating habits, using the correct food supplements, following suitable stress management techniques and ensuring spiritual growth, as well as exercising regularly, we could all improve our own lives and those of others. This would enable us to lead happy, fulfilled and healthy lives. Internally our physiological and biochemical balance would be restored to normal (reaching homeostasis) and we would notice the difference in our body, emotions, mind and soul.

Research increasingly confirms that a change in lifestyle is the single most important adjustment that we need to make to address health problems:

1. Our eating habits must change to a more natural, whole-food diet that contains plenty of fresh fruit and vegetables, pulses, seeds, nuts and wholegrain products. Reduce your intake of red meat and eat fish and poultry in moderation. The food pyramid provides a general guideline for our daily requirements. It has been proved conclusively that the symptoms of all the chronic diseases and allergies benefit from a change in eating habits.

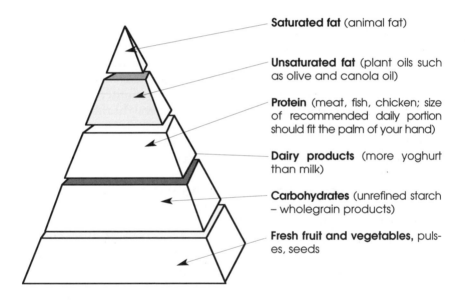

Saturated fat (animal fat)

Unsaturated fat (plant oils such as olive and canola oil)

Protein (meat, fish, chicken; size of recommended daily portion should fit the palm of your hand)

Dairy products (more yoghurt than milk)

Carbohydrates (unrefined starch – wholegrain products)

Fresh fruit and vegetables, pulses, seeds

2. The correct food supplements are essential in the hectic and stressful lives we live today. The main part of this book is devoted to the topic of micronutrients and the need to supplement the daily diet because there is so much confusion, controversy and uncertainty surrounding these issues. Is it necessary to take food supplements or not? Which supplements and what quantities do individuals need for their particular circumstances?

3. Herbs are plants with healing properties that can improve our health and wellbeing and restore function to the systems of the body. Although herbs are natural, it is not always safe to take them together with ordinary prescription medicine. The increased interest in the use of medicinal herbs does not mean that we always understand exactly how they work. Herbal medicine is well integrated into Eastern medicine, both orthodox and complementary. However, it is still comparatively new to Western medical doctors and researchers. There is little real expertise and knowledge on herbal medicine – especially when herbs are taken together with conventional medicine.

   Too little research has been done on the interaction of the various prescription medicines with each other. The pharmaceutical industry is well regulated, but there is not enough information and research on the interaction of prescription drugs with each other – let alone the interaction between prescription drugs and herbs.

   Herbs are combinations of many ingredients. Do not randomly mix herbs with over-the-counter and prescription medication. If you are uncertain, consult someone who is knowledgeable on herbal remedies as well as prescription and over-the-counter drugs. Most herbs are quite harmless and improve general health. However, everyone has a unique psychological, emotional, mental and physical make-up. You will need to use and experiment with the herbs recommended for your condition. If they don't work for you, try something else.

   This book concentrates mainly on herbs that are well researched in the West and that are regularly prescribed by medical doctors trained in complementary or alternative therapies. The recommended dosages are based on the use of single ingredients. **When using combinations of micronutrients, the dosages can be reduced considerably.** Remember that all micronutrients work together synergistically and that less of each ingredient is needed in a combination because together they support each other's functions.

4. Increasingly there is reason to believe that stress lies at the root of most modern diseases. This is why two chapters deal with the role of stress in the body, facts on positive and negative stress and practical ways to manage stress.

5. Regular exercise is essential for a healthy body and mind. Most people are physically able to exercise regularly. It is not necessary to buy expensive sports equipment or join a health club. Most people enjoy walking. Walking is cheap, sociable and allows us to appreciate

nature. Thirty minutes of walking four times a week is sufficient exercise for most people.

Let us once again combine the art of healing with the science of medicine.

1 The role of stress in the body

Stress is a reaction to something or someone that is experienced by the individual via the senses as stressful to the body. What or who-ever causes the stress reaction is called the stressor.

We all need a certain amount of stress to be able to live. In fact, we would all die without it. Stress keeps us going. It helps us to achieve, work, excel and strive towards growth and fulfilment in different fields. However, it is important for us to remain in the positive stress phase by balancing periods of stress with regular healing phases of rest and relaxation.

Constant, unbalanced and chronic stress must be avoided or managed. It is this form of stress, tension and anxiety that has probably become the most common and serious problem of our time. It affects all the functions of our mind and body. Our entire being is involved in the daily stress of living. Stress affects every aspect of our lives and it is important for us to know how to change our attitude so that we can choose not to react subjectively to certain situations. We are not always able to avoid stressful situations, which is why we should learn how to cope with them. We can only manage and change the way we react to a specific stressor.

Does this sound easier said than done? Read the whole chapter before you decide.

Stress is the way an individual reacts physiologically, psychologically, emotionally and behaviourally in order to adapt, change and regain equilibrium in response to internal and external pressure.

A stressor trigger is any situation, person, object or event that an individual experiences as stressful. The result is a stress reaction experienced by the entire body and mind. Stressors can vary significantly. Stress can be caused psychologically after an attack, accident or rape. This leads to post-traumatic stress disorder which usually needs treatment by specialists trained in cognitive behavioural therapy. Examples of physical stressors include noise, pollution, low blood sugar levels (hypoglycaemia) and environmental temperature. Stress can also have causes that are founded on emotional and mental factors such as problems in a relationship, frustration, anger, revenge, antagonism, prejudice, fear, overwork and taking on too much (trying to do too much or to please everyone). Imagination and anticipation of bad or unpleasant things cause most of our stress reactions.

The stress reaction is really a fear reaction. We all experience situations or things which frighten us and lead to stress. These are usually very personal and unique to each individual. This is why each of us is responsible for changing our own perceptions.

Stress is a genetically inherent reaction or process to ensure the survival of the human species and that of all other living organisms (plants and animals). It is called the fight or flight reaction. In prehistoric times the early humans had either to confront the danger and fight, or take to their heels.

Humans today react in the same way. We may not always have to cope with the same direct physical threats that our ancestors had to face and we do not have the same physical release of fight or flight. Instead we suffer from psychological stress caused by fear (emotion). Whether the fear is real or imaginary, we have the same stress reaction. The body and the mind, however, cannot always distinguish between a real threat to our lives and an imagined threat created in our minds. Increase your awareness of your surroundings so that you are better able to sense real danger and to put it in perspective. This will enable you to respond more appropriately to real danger, based on your inner instinct for survival (intuition) instead of being paralysed by fear.

The human body constantly maintains an internal balance and stability (homeostasis). We depend on this process for optimal health and wellbeing. The body responds to stress through a complicated series of biochemical reactions involving all the systems of the body. After the stress reaction, the balance must be restored so that the normal bodily functions can continue. If this does not happen, various organs and systems will become depleted.

The stress reaction

What happens in the body during a stress reaction? Why is it important for this reaction to be controlled?

Our nervous system is the same as that of our prehistoric ancestors. But we are more advanced intellectually and emotionally and should develop the insight to cope better with stress. Our external environment and inner thought processes need not toss us about like a cork on stormy seas. If we cope with our stress in the correct way, we can utilise and apply the stress reaction for its actual purpose – to ensure our survival.

Diagram 1: The physiology of stress – a representation of the stress reaction and its effect on the body

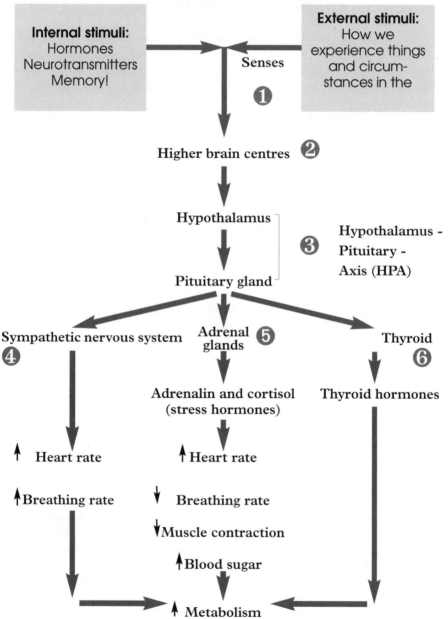

Our brains and nervous systems are not able to distinguish between real physical danger and a psychological feeling of danger. The body interprets real and imaginary messages of fear in the same way and the same stress reaction occurs.

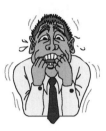

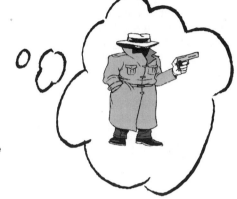

Thoughts in the mind can cause a physical stress reaction in the whole body.

The effect of stress on the body

All stress-related reactions cause a subjective perception or awareness which is transmitted via the ❶ senses (hearing, sight, smell, touch, taste, as well as the non-physical senses such as intuition and electromagnetic fields) ❷ to the higher centres) in the brain cortex.

❶ Senses (perceptual awareness)

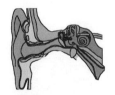

e.g. hearing and sight

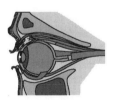

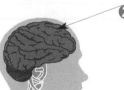

❷ Higher centres in the brain cortex

❸ Hypothalamus, pituitary axis (situated deep in the centre of the brain between the two hemispheres)

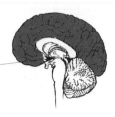

From the ❸ hypothalamus, pituitary gland and brain stem (the brain centre in early reptiles), messages are transmitted by the neurotransmitters in the nervous system and hormones in the blood to:

❹ The sympathetic part of the nervous system where stress causes a racing heart, shortness of breath and increased metabolism.

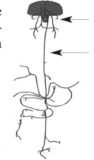

Brain where pituitary gland is situated

Messages go via the sympathetic nervous system to the whole body including the heart, lungs, muscles and skin.

❺ The adrenal glands (above the two kidneys) which activate the secretion of the stress hormones, cortisol, adrenalin and noradrenaline. These important hormones cause a racing heart, rapid breathing, muscle contractions, stimulation of the bladder wall, high blood sugar levels and increased metabolism. They stimulate the skin to perspire more in order to bring down the higher temperature caused by an increase in metabolism. At the same time the urogenital, digestive and immune systems are suppressed because these systems are not needed in the stress reaction.

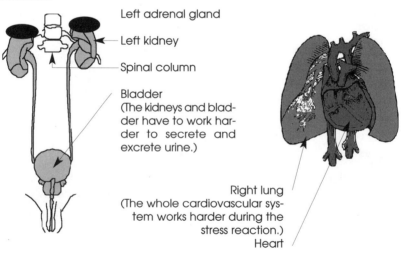

Left adrenal gland

Left kidney

Spinal column

Bladder
(The kidneys and bladder have to work harder to secrete and excrete urine.)

Right lung
(The whole cardiovascular system works harder during the stress reaction.)
Heart

⑥ The thyroid gland which secretes thyroid hormones which in turn increase the metabolism.

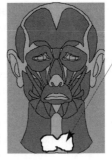

. Thyroid excretes T3 and T4 hormones which accelerate the metabolism of the whole body.

It is clear that the whole body is involved in the stress reaction:

- The senses, brain cortex, hypothalamus and pituitary gland set the reaction in motion and control it.
- The whole endocrine system, represented by the hormones in the blood, actively controls the activities of all the organs during stress. The cardiovascular system, including the heart, lungs and blood vessels, have to work hard to ensure that every cell is supplied with enough oxygen and blood sugar to provide energy. The muscles, joints and ligaments of the musculoskeletal system are all ready for the fight or flight response. The kidneys and bladder actively form more concentrated urine (kidneys) and excrete it (bladder). The liver and pancreas must ensure that there is enough blood sugar to provide energy for all these processes to take place.
- The skin has a twofold involvement in the stress reaction: the increased metabolism stimulates it to excrete more sweat to prevent the body from overheating while simultaneously the blood is rerouted from the skin to the more vital stress systems such as the heart, lungs and muscles. The skin gets less blood during the stress reaction and waste products can easily accumulate.
- The blood supply to the digestive tract is reduced as the digestive process is not immediately essential to the stress reaction.

It is now clear why uncontrolled stress or stress which is not managed properly (or managed at all) has been identified as the underlying catalyst behind many diseases of our time.

Some examples

A person has a family history of a genetic defect in the cardiovascular or respiratory system. The person is also a great worrier and workaholic. Tension builds up; the person always expects the worst, blames others for everything that goes wrong, has angry outbursts and resents people for different reasons. The inevitable result is that the person will develop high blood pressure (hypertension) or asthma, chronic bronchitis or even lung cancer. This person is probably a smoker to 'relieve the tension', does little or no exercise and has an unhealthy diet. All these factors contribute to the disease process, which is merely a physical symptom or sign of a deeper problem. Simply keeping the blood pressure down with medication will not help. The blood pressure medication will probably cause side effects which will lead to other problems that will need to be treated with more medication – a vicious circle develops.

A family history of **skin problems** (with all the above factors) may manifest as eczema, flare-ups of psoriasis and severe acne.

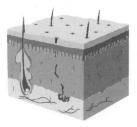

The skin receives contrasting messages during the stress reaction: Perspiration (sweat production) must increase, but blood supply to parts of the skin is reduced. The result is skin complaints such as eczema, psoriasis or acne.

A genetic problem in the **nervous system,** together with many years of tension, suppressed emotions and negative feelings can lead to depression, anxiety poor concentration and even Alzheimer's disease.

Digestive tract: Spastic colon (irritable bowel syndrome), gastritis, ulcers – even ulcerative colitis and Crohn's disease have a significant stress and family history component.

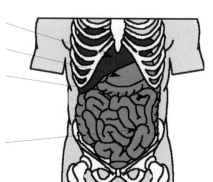

Liver

Stomach: gastritis, ulcers

Colon: spastic colon, ulcerative colitis, diarrhoea or constipation

Small intestines: poor digestion, food intolerance, Crohn's disease

Endocrine system: An overactive or underactive thyroid and an imbalance in the adrenal glands can result in a weakened immune system, leading to chronic infections or even cancer. The immune system is the first system in the body to indicate if there has been too much stress over too long a period. If you constantly suffer from infections and fever blisters, listen to your body and slow down. The secretion of insulin by the pancreas can be disrupted, leading to hypoglycaemia (low blood sugar) or diabetes. In people who already have diabetes, it can be aggravated or become uncontrollable.

Musculoskeletal system: Arthritis in any form, muscular pain, muscle spasms, backache, gout, etc.

Urogenital system: Overstimulation of the kidneys and bladder can lead to symptoms such as weakened bladder control, infections, incontinence and the urge to urinate at night. Severe menopausal symptoms, premenstrual syndrome (PMS), irregular menstruation, low libido and infertility are problems where poor stress management or too much stress plays an important role.

In the past high blood pressure, cancer, chronic fatigue (yuppy flu or ME), high cholesterol and similar ailments were not nearly as common as they are today. Family history and the stress reaction have not changed. But our ancestors did not have to face the relentless mental stress, the technologically challenging, computer-driven endless workday we have today (using the Internet, cellular phone, laptops even on holiday); nor did they lack physical activity to give expression to the fight or flight reaction.

The stress reaction is identical to the reaction of prehistoric humans and our ancestors. The difference is that prehistoric humans had an immediate physical outlet; so the reaction was short lived. The person would get a fright, fight or take flight and then lie down to sleep. In the simpler stages of human evolution people were thus better equipped to cope with stress. We have progressed intellectually and stress is created mainly in our minds, where it is internalised and developed further. However, unlike early humankind we are intellectually advanced enough to know how to control our thoughts and emotions. We can utilise our stress reactions positively to the benefit of our mental, emotional and physical wellbeing.

Stress is thus a primitive reaction in a modern society. Short-term exposure to stress, such as a near accident, allows the body to return to normal very quickly. This is why you feel drained after a big shock. Sleep is an excellent method that the parasympathetic nervous system uses to restore balance to the sympathetic nervous system (that sets off the stress reaction).

Severe constant stress eventually results in negative stress and exhaustion or disease and symptoms of chronic fatigue, constant niggling infections, depression, headaches and all the chronic diseases already mentioned. The weak links in the biochemical chains (existing genetic or family weakness that determines the system manifestation) are the first to collapse and break.

Our goal is to aim for a positive stress phase. Signs of this are:

- Increased creativity – not only in making or creating things, but also in developing new ways to solve problems or finding better ways of doing things.
- Increased productivity at work and on a personal level.
- A general feeling of wellbeing, happiness and joy – which is how we should feel. It is our birthright to lead happy, fulfilled lives during our physical sojourn on earth.
- An immune system that functions optimally, with an increased resistance to infections and cancer. Even if you're surrounded by people with all kinds of germs, you simply don't become ill. People in remission from cancer come to realise what is important to them in life and experience an inner growth and development, which often leads to physical healing. Even people who eventually die of cancer gain an awareness of the temporary nature of the physical body as opposed to the soul that lives forever. This realisation that the spirit lives on leads to a feeling of inner peace, happiness and wellbeing.

The warning signs for a negative stress phase are:

- Reduced productivity and creativity: Nothing works the way it should. Everything is too much for you. You cannot find the solutions to problems. You are unable to concentrate or remember things. Depression starts in much the same way.
- A reduced feeling of wellbeing, joy and happiness: You no longer enjoy anything. You don't look forward to anything. Everything is a burden. These symptoms can be precursors to depression unless you take the necessary precautions timeously.
- All sorts of unfortunate things happen to you. You become so preoccupied with the daily stress of living that you are unable to focus or

concentrate. This leads to car accidents; you drop and break things or lose them. You cut yourself or break an arm.

- You start avoiding social contact. Avoiding people for long periods of time is also a sign of depression. Remember that socialising is one of the basic human needs.
- Reduced resistance: Your immune system functions poorly and you suffer from colds, flu, allergies, autoimmune diseases, chronic fatigue, anxiety attacks and all the diseases already mentioned – unless you take the necessary steps to restore your equilibrium.
- Your organs and systems start to fail and physical disease processes start.
- The ageing process accelerates because of the increased metabolism associated with uncontrolled stress. Free radicals and other waste products accumulate and cell activity deteriorates, resulting in premature ageing. (See p. 59.)

In conclusion

Stress-related health problems would include angina, asthma, autoimmune diseases (such as rheumatoid arthritis, lupus, multiple sclerosis, ulcerative colitis and psoriasis), cancer, cardiovascular diseases, colds, depression, substance abuse, diabetes (especially type 2), headaches, high blood pressure, immune suppression, AIDS, spastic colon (irritable bowel syndrome), menstrual disorders, premenstrual tension and ulcers.

Once we realise that we are to a large extent responsible for our own disease processes (even though it happens unconsciously), it is counterproductive to develop a guilty conscience – that would only lead to further stress! The realisation should help you take control of your healing process. If something doesn't work, change it or change your attitude. If you unconsciously played a role in creating your illness, the realisation that you can also play a role in your healing process is very empowering.

Stress is very personal, but it is also a sociological and corporate problem. Think of how many hours at work are lost because of diseases, high blood pressure and heart attacks. Think of a person's quality of life after a heart attack or stroke with partial recovery. Think of the hospital bills. Think of the effect on young children and the family if a parent dies of a stress-related disease. Let's do something about it!

2 Practical stress management techniques

Stress management improves the function of the cardiovascular system, decreases the secretion of the stress hormones (adrenalin, noradrenaline and cortisol), improves the absorption of oxygen in the cells of the body, leads to an improved self-image and a feeling of wellbeing, relieves the symptoms of depression, anxiety and tension, and raises energy levels.

The twelve-point stress management plan for a happier and healthier life

Apply the following 12 life-enhancing points in your life and see how the quality of your life improves.

1 Getting to know yourself and diagnosing negative stress

Getting to know yourself is an essential part of successful stress management. You begin to realise that you have control over how you experience the things within you and around you. Even if you have inherited your grandmother's sensitive disposition, as you've been told repeatedly since you were a child, you can decide *today* to change your attitude to life. We all have the capacity to change if we really want to. It could take a while; personality traits have become ingrained over a lifetime – you can't expect to change overnight.

Read positive, constructive and informative books. Broaden your horizon. Break the years of self-imposed limitations and chains that have crippled your spiritual growth and development. Don't allow anyone or anything the power to run your life for you. You have to decide who or what is able to influence you positively.

Accept and love yourself. Look at yourself in the mirror when you get up in the morning. Before you brush your hair, wash your face or brush your teeth, look at yourself and say, 'Hello, gorgeous, I love you.'

Go on, try it! It works!

Talk to people. Many of us have had similar experiences in our lives. Ask for advice and you will soon realise that you are not alone. If you are having difficulty processing events, feelings and fears from the past, and leaving them behind, seek professional psychological help.

Some hints and thoughts on psychotherapy

It is no good tormenting yourself for years about things which happened in the past with associated feelings of guilt, fear, revenge, hatred and criticism of yourself and others. Grow and move beyond these things. Leave negative feelings where they belong – in the past – and go on with the present. It's all you have! Make an appointment to consult someone who specialises in cognitive behavioural or analytical therapy.

A psychotherapist tries to help individuals to recover their self-worth. The patient is brought back to intuitive self-knowledge about the really important and valuable things in their lives.

We are inclined to assess value and quality with materialistic guidelines in rands and cents or in scientifically measurable quantities. We want things to be cost effective, with results pre-determined and calculated. We must change our technological, analytical, typically Western left-brain thinking to a more balanced perception of the really important things in life – love, happiness, joy, creativity-right-brain activities. We are all subconsciously looking for these things, but in the wrong places. We will never find them in material things, other people, drugs, alcohol or any other external substances. They can only be found within ourselves. Happiness is our birthright and it lies within our soul.

Most people start psychotherapy with a deep feeling of ignorance and uncertainty about their own worth. Too little value has been attached to their own inner being. What they are saying is: I need and deserve attention; I have a purpose and goal to achieve on earth; I am valuable. This is a sincere conviction, even if at first it is hidden by the layers that the ego has woven around the soul. Such a person is mainly aware of overwhelming feelings of uselessness, grief, sadness, pain, unhappiness, rage, confusion and despair.

But the resilience of the human spirit is boundless. Wellbeing is not just an absence of the symptoms of disease. It is a deep-seated inner feeling of happiness, joy, satisfaction and peace. As soon as you realise this, you know that all these feelings are waiting for you, deep within yourself and in your soul.

2 Positive thinking and attitude

Even if it is sometimes difficult to remain positive, remember the saying, 'Fake it until you make it.' If you teach yourself to appear positive for long enough, eventually being positive will become part of your personality.

Research shows that positive, optimistic people have a better immune function. They are thus better able to fight disease and cancer. Negative emotions are found to have a strong effect on the body's immune system via the neurotransmitters. In the short term this leads to recurrent, niggling infections and over the longer term to autoimmune diseases (where the body attacks its own cells), cancer, chronic diseases and premature ageing. Rage, hatred and cynicism lead to disease, fear and death.

In any situation you can choose how you are going to react. You have to live through the bad things that happen to you in life. You must experience them, grieve them, learn from them and become wiser. You should not suppress your emotions; nor should you spend the rest of your life reliving these events and moping about them. They are in the past and cannot be changed. Your attitude and way of thinking are the only things that can change. The only failure in life is not having tried.

> **Shakespeare:** Things are rarely good or bad, but our thinking makes it so!
>
> **Carl Jung:** It all depends on how we look at things, and not on how they are in themselves.
>
> **Victor E. Frankl** (written in a German concentration camp during the Second World War): Everything can be taken from a man but one thing: the last of the human freedoms – to choose one's attitude in any given set of circumstances, to choose one's own way.

You are not a victim!

Avoid negative people or help them to become more positive. Don't allow people or things to upset you. You allow the person, situation or event to cause you stress. However simple this advice may seem, it is not easy to follow. It takes practice before you realise that you can choose how to react and before it becomes part of your new personality.

Don't allow your thoughts to dwell on negative things from the past or worry all the time about what might happen in the future. Your fears and concerns can do nothing to change the situation. Don't deny or suppress these thoughts; just observe them objectively, move beyond them and focus on pleasant things. You can choose to act in this way.

Stress, adversity and change teach us more about ourselves and motivate us to inner growth and greater awareness of ourselves and our environment.

There is a positive side to everything. It can take years to see things in this way, but traumatic events will often guide you to a new life and new way of thinking full of growth and development. Think of half a glass of water as half full and not half empty!

Many of us have chosen unconsciously to grow and develop through taking the difficult course, suffering and struggling. It is not necessary to learn in this way. We can also choose to grow consciously through the good and positive things in life.

We are daily exposed to crime. This is a good example of how fear, anxiety, guilt, despair and hatred constantly evoke the fight or flight reaction, which has to be processed and balanced.

Many South African men have been brought up with the idea that they should suppress all their emotions and they find it difficult to cope in South Africa today. Every man lives with the thought that he and his family are potential targets of criminal activities. We all have to deal with feelings of helplessness and hatred. As already mentioned, we are too attached to our material possessions and the loss of them causes intense shock and anxiety.

Emotionally, women tend to cope with this type of trauma better than men. Society allows women to give expression to a wide range of emotions. The socially acceptable reaction (however) for men is aggression and rage – certainly not heartache, uncertainty, vulnerability, fear and an overwhelming feeling of helplessness.

We all have to learn to cope with this stressor. We cannot suddenly change it; we can't really move house or move to another country; we can't run away; we can't attack the aggressor. We have to find the answer within ourselves.

What is important is that people should talk to one another. Partners should communicate their feelings to each other. Relationships with other people create a safe, confidential space for sharing feelings.

Good things can develop from bad experiences. People are reaching out to one another again. Couples are learning to talk to each other, men are discovering that it is normal to feel uncertain, scared and helpless. This is often a stimulus for spiritual growth and an awareness of the important things in life. People sometimes decide to realise life-long dreams or try a new job. How you tackle a situation is your choice.

We must become more alert and learn to spot signs of danger in the neighbourhood. Criminals don't just appear from nowhere. If we were less concerned about tomorrow and less regretful about yesterday, we would be better able to focus on the present and not operate in a state of unawareness of our surroundings. This would enable us to use the fight or flight reaction for the purpose for which it was created.

By taking control of how you utilise your fear reaction, you can change from being a victim to being in control of a situation.

Today's society is generally very negative, but we must start the healing process. We cannot wait for the government or the police service to do everything. Emphasise the power of love, rather than the power of hate. South Africa is in a period of transition which will lead to the rebirth of a more tolerant and balanced society – perhaps in our lifetime, perhaps not. It is difficult to see the light when it's still dark. Remember, that darkness is neither an entity nor a reality – it is only a place where the light is absent. There is a deep feeling of mutual respect and dignity among most of the people in our country. Let us build on that feeling!

3 Wholesome nutrition, correct supplementation and gentle exercise

The mind and soul cannot soar, dream or grow if the body does not function at peak metabolic performance level. You must eat wholesome, unrefined ('living'), food to keep your body in peak condition. This includes a daily intake of a variety of vegetables, fruit, pulses, seeds, wholegrain products and other unrefined carbohydrates. Restrict your intake of animal fats and other saturated fats such as butter, fatty meat, margarine, fried foods, cakes, chocolate and junk food. Make sure that you consume enough mono- and polyunsaturated fats as a source of omega-3 and omega-6 essential fatty acids. Get your daily fat requirement in the form of oily fish such as salmon, trout, sardines, and mackerel, as well as olive oil, canola oil and linseed oil (flax oil). (Consult Chapter 9 on essential fatty acids.)

Use food supplements every day. All the biochemical reactions in the body are activated, catalised and maintained by enzymes. All the metabolic processes depend on enzymes. Enzymes need support from vitamins and minerals with amino acids and fatty acids to function optimally.

The stress reaction, particularly chronic stress, results in a very active metabolism. This places huge demands on the enzymes, which then need more support from vitamins, minerals, fatty acids and amino acids. It is very difficult to maintain this through your daily dietary intake alone. Food supplementation is thus essential. Supplements provide support for the active production of stress hormones (adrenalin, noradrenaline and cortisol) by the adrenal cortex. They boost the nervous and endocrine systems. Medicinal herbs reduce the damage of free radicals and prevent physical and mental exhaustion.

During times of accelerated metabolism, lots of free radicals are formed. These can accumulate in the cells and eventually cause damage. We need more antioxidants such as vitamins A, C and E as well as the minerals zinc, selenium and copper to limit the damage. It is extremely difficult to provide these needs from diet alone. Marginal deficiencies of micronutrients in the presence of persistent stress play a major role in the onset of almost all chronic diseases. (Consult Chapters 4 and 5 on food supplements and antioxidants.)

Don't overlook the healing properties of herbs. Most medicinal herbs are intended for human consumption to ensure good health. Use them in the preparation of food, as aromatic fragrances for your home, as a preventive health measure and as an excellent mild method of treating almost any form of disease. Consult a good book on herbs for details. Start with a few basic herbs: ginger, cinnamon, sage, basil, thyme, rosemary, geranium, lavender, neroli, aloe, calendula, lemon balm and camomile.

Some medicinal herbs such as ginseng are adaptogens – they can adapt themselves in the body and move to any cell to restore specific functions within the cell as required. The active ingredients in the herbs penetrate the cell membrane, often moving right into the nucleus and from there into the deoxyribonucleic acid (DNA), the genetic nucleus material of the cell. This can subtly and gently improve the functioning of the secretion of hormones and the transfer of messages in the nervous system. Adaptogens promote the ability of the body to resist stressors. They therefore assist the body in coping with stress.

Well-known adaptogens are Asian, True or Chinese ginseng (*Panax ginseng*), American ginseng (*Panax quinquefolius*), Siberian ginseng (*Eleutherococcus senticosus*), liquorice or glycyrrhiza root (*Glycyrrhiza alba*), schisandra, astragalus and Reishi, Shiitake and Maitaki mushrooms. Almost all medicinal herbs are adaptogens. Make sure that the products you use are from a reliable and reputable source.

Adaptogens help the body to cope with stress by providing antioxidant activity, protecting the liver; improving blood sugar metabolism; reducing the craving for alcohol or sweetness; improving immunity and resistance; energy and stamina; improving muscle tone; decreasing fatigue; accelerating recovery after diseases and operations; improving focus and concentration; decreasing anxiety; improving sleeping patterns, motivation and productivity; providing a feeling of pleasure, a better state of mind and a general balance in the whole physiology.

Don't use herbal preparations haphazardly without knowing something about them. Herbs can be very potent and harmful in the wrong hands. Consult an expert or an authoritative book on herbs.

Good nutrition, the correct food supplements and regular use of herbs balance our physiology. Correct nutrition reaches the very essence of our being. Remember, we become what we eat. All our food is broken down into its basic elements and becomes part of every cell, hormone and neurotransmitter in our body.

A good place to start to make us more aware of our bodies, minds and souls and the control we have over our own health and wellbeing is by becoming aware of our food intake and by using supplements.

Physical activity in the form of moderate, gentle exercise is important for balance in the nervous system. It meets the need for a physical outlet for the fight or flight stress reaction. Exercise strengthens your state of mind and results in increased intellectual alertness and better concentration.

Regular exercise results in a measurable increase in the neurotransmitters in the brain (such as serotonin), responsible for a feeling of wellbeing and pleasure. Exercise is also an excellent way of alleviating depression.

4 Time management, planning and organisation

Get your priorities right. Make a list of the things you have to do and arrange them in order of importance or urgency. Then start with the first item. Just sitting down and getting started on a huge job is encouraging in itself. You have taken control of the situation and it becomes manageable. If you keep worrying about how you will ever finish, you despair before you even begin.

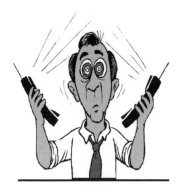

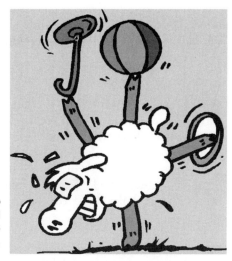

Draw up a list of priorities and say **No** to things involving too much work and responsibility. Then you won't give up in despair before you've even begun.

Learn to say 'No'! Women often feel obliged to agree to take on more and more things to please other people. Afterwards they are sorry and do the job with a feeling of resentment. When it comes to charity work, realise that you can choose what kind of contribution to make. If you hate baking cakes, don't agree to bake a cake for the church fête. Offer to arrange flowers if you enjoy doing that more. Utilise your talents and preferences.

Once you have made a decision, stick to it. Don't develop feelings of guilt or torment yourself. You've said 'No' – don't change your mind. Trust your intuition and instinct when it tries to protect you from taking on too much. Don't allow people to manipulate you. It will only aggravate your stress problem. When you feel that you are really not able to take on something, try saying 'No' just once and feel the sense of self-empowerment.

5 Time for relaxation

Everyone should set aside some time every day to sit back, breathe deeply, relax and enjoy the moment. This helps us to focus on the present.

Use techniques that focus your attention on the here and now. Choose what seems right for you. Don't judge the choices others make. Do what feels right for you and remember that mastering any new technique takes time and practice.

Consider one of these suggestions: Listen to relaxing music or take music appreciation classes, dance to the rhythm of mood music or try self-hypnosis and positive reinforcement. (Consult the list of references at the back of the book.) Enlist for a course in practical philosophy. Take pottery or painting lessons. Join a support group or an interest group such as a book club or start your own group. Attending meditation sessions is an excellent way of eliciting the relaxation response. There are various kinds of meditation techniques. Choose one that you feel comfortable with. Remember that the Christian and all other religions have a rich history of meditation – with the emergence of Calvinism and the modern mind-set we seem to have lost it along the way. Prayer is also a form of meditation. Prayer is a means of communicating with God. Meditation enables God to communicate with you from within the silence of your soul.

Dr Herbert Benson wrote a book called *Timeless Healing.* I strongly recommend Benson's relaxation response. He is a cardiologist associated with the Harvard Medical School and chief of Behavioural Medicine at the New England Deaconess Hospital. He has done research on meditation – from yoga, Hindu, Sufism, Judaism and Zen to the Christian form of meditation. He has found that the common objective of all these divergent cultural techniques is the evocation of a quiet mind and a peaceful heart that manifests in a healthy body, a feeling of wellbeing and spiritual growth. He calls this technique the relaxation response. He has lifted the mystical veil surrounding meditation from the mists of Western ignorance. Don't allow prejudices and fears to prevent you from utilising the easily attainable and scientifically proven advantages of meditation.

You may wonder how such a simple technique can benefit your mind and body to such an extent. Try it for ten minutes morning and evening for two weeks and then decide if it is worthwhile. You remain aware of your surroundings throughout and in complete control of the situation.

Requirements

- Choose a quiet peaceful area at home or in the office, a scenic spot outdoors or any other place where there is no noise or disturbance.
- Find a technique for calming down your frantic thoughts ('monkey

chatter') and guiding them beyond the usual, logical, distracting, thought processes and worries. This is similar to using a mantra in Eastern meditation techniques. Choose a one- or two-syllable word with a low tonality and repeat it loudly or softly in a calm tone of voice. Good examples are loving, sun, moon, one, tree, ground, water, sea, god.

- Be passive. Try not to focus on how well or how badly you are doing the exercise or whether you are achieving the desired reaction. Simply observe your thoughts, let them pass and concentrate on repeating the word you have chosen.
- Get into a comfortable position so that you can relax physically and mentally. You should not be aware of any tension in your muscles or anywhere else in your body. Sit in a comfortable chair which supports your back and head well. You can also lie on your bed. If you fall asleep, that's fine. Sleep is excellent for restoring balance in the body and mind by counteracting the stress reaction.

How to relax

- Sit comfortably in a quiet place.
- Close your eyes.
- Breathe deeply. Take a deep breath to the count of four while pushing your stomach muscles out (yes, push *out*). Hold the breath for six counts and then blow out the air hard and fast. Repeat this five times.
- Relax all your muscles. Start with your toes, then move to your feet, ankles, calves, thighs, buttocks, stomach, chest, shoulders, arms, hands, fingers, neck and head. Feel the tension draining away. Focus on any tension that you still feel and let it go.
- While you are quietly breathing in and out, repeat your word to yourself, either softly or out loud. If your attention wanders, quietly bring your thoughts back to your word and repeat it again. Don't get angry with yourself for being unable to concentrate.
- Do this exercise for ten to 20 minutes every day. Don't set an alarm clock. Look at the clock after a while. Open your eyes slowly, become aware of your surroundings, wiggle your toes and enjoy the feeling of peace, calm and contentment.

Other techniques

- If you have more time, you can continue with the following technique while you are in a relaxed condition: Picture yourself in a garden that you've been in before. It is a beautiful, peaceful place. Sit there and use all your senses to visualise your surroundings in your mind's eye. Look at all the things around you. Use your ears, nose, skin and tongue. Messages may come to you from your unconscious in the shape of people, angels, etc. Listen to them and write them down after the exercise. You will often find unexpected solutions to problems in this way.
- Keep a dream diary next to your bed. As soon as you wake up, either during the night or in the morning, write down your dreams. You will become more aware of your dreams and the symbolic messages that come from your unconscious through your dreams.

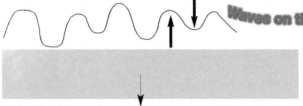

Waves on the surface of the ocean

The deepest part of the ocean where it is calm and peaceful

- Think of your thoughts as the waves on the surface of the ocean. They go up and down as your mood, feelings, emotions and memory dictate. The deeper part of the ocean is quiet, calm and peaceful. This is the part of yourself that you can access voluntarily at any time through meditation, visualisation, deep breathing, guided imagery and prayer. By diving into the depths of your soul, you can observe your external life and cope better with it.
- Remember that learning a new habit like meditation may take time. Do it regularly every day. You will soon see the results.
- Enjoy a long relaxing bath. Close the doors and disconnect the phone. Light a candle and switch off the lights. Add a few drops of aromatherapy oil to the water (camomile, neroli, lavender or sandalwood). Play peaceful music and enjoy a glass of wine while you are in the bath. There are few things with such an immediate positive relaxing effect. Try it tonight!

All these relaxation techniques and ideas help to remove the greatest stumbling blocks on the road to human happiness, namely anxiety and fear.

6 Balance right and left brain activities

The left brain is responsible for our analytical, rational, logical and sequential thinking abilities. Western culture and our educational and working environment place considerable emphasis on left brain function.

The right brain controls our emotions, intuition, visualisation skills, music appreciation abilities and creativity. Most people completely deny this fundamental aspect of being human. This results in an imbalance, with the result that our ability to cope with stress is severely curtailed.

Make time every day for right brain activities. Choose something you enjoy. There are many examples such as pottery, painting, gardening, flower arranging, knitting, sewing, writing children's stories, poetry or other stories. Allow your imagination free reign! It does not matter how good or bad you think you are at these activities, just do it for the enjoyment thereof.

Learn to appreciate your emotions. Pay attention to your intuitive feelings about things that happen or are said. We tend to suppress these feelings – often to our great regret. How many times do you feel you can't trust someone? You suppress this inner 'guardian angel', only to realise later that you should have paid more attention. Learn to do things because they 'feel' right. The more you use your right brain, the more actively it will change and influence your life for the better.

Doing altruistic acts for other people is wonderful for our stress levels and encourages us to connect with reality. Expressions of love and sociability are the most basic human needs. The soul has a need for compassion and genuineness.

Give thanks every day for all the good things that have happened that day. Make a mental list of all the positive things. When we realise how much we have to be thankful for, we create an aura of abundance. People concentrate so much on the negative things that they often forget to be grateful for the things they do have.

7 Tolerance, flexibility and adaptability

Learn to go with the flow. Don't always try swimming up-stream and changing everything. Life is not like that. Things are seldom as perfect as you would like them to be. Learning to accept situations and not allowing them to upset you is excellent stress management. Remember that change is the only constant factor in life!

Don't be rigid and disapproving. Accept other people and their ideas. You will never change someone else by insisting that you and your opinions and convictions are the only right ones. We shouldn't be so arrogant as to think that we know all the answers and the right way. Accept other people as they are and learn from them. Each of us has a path to follow in life. By changing your perceptions you will get rid of an enormous amount of frustration, rage and repressed anxiety.

If you pass judgement on other people and their ideas and culture, you are only harming your own soul and disturbing your own peace of mind. Read books to help you to change your perspective on life.

8 Enthusiasm as a permanent part of who you are

The word enthusiasm comes from the ancient Greek, *entheos*, inspired (en- = in and -thios = god). Enthusiasm is very infectious. If you learn how to become excited about things, you will seldom be depressed or stressed for long.

Enjoy what you do and do it to the best of your ability. If you are convinced that what you are doing is right for you and that you are enjoying it, the sense of wellbeing you feel will became quite obvious to yourself and others.

9 Sense of humour

Most things in life have a funny side – always try to look for it. Laughter removes all feelings of stress. People who laugh a lot have an excellent immune system and seldom get sick. Their stress threshold is also high so that few things can upset them and make them tense. The ability to laugh is a natural human characteristic.

Force yourself to smile, even if you don't feel like it. You will soon learn to smile more easily and notice a difference in your quality of life.

Look at yourself in the mirror, smile at yourself and say, 'You gorgeous thing, I love you.'

As soon as you start projecting a lively happy personality, you will make it your own. People are naturally attracted to happy people.

10 Wisdom

Stress management is a philosophy of life. You have to develop the inner wisdom to stop searching for instant solutions outside your own soul. Learn to look inwards – then you won't keep looking for solutions and excuses from outside. You will also stop blaming others for everything that goes wrong in your life.

Try to stop asking why things happen. We cannot be expected to know everything. What happens to us as individuals is a small speck in the context of the universal spectrum. We can only experience what life offers us and develop our spiritual knowledge that the body is temporary, but that the spirit and soul live forever. This inner knowledge will help us to continue along the joyful path that is our birthright.

This prayer has stood the test of time: O God, give me the strength to change the things I can, the patience to accept the things I cannot change and the wisdom to know the difference.

11 Spiritual nourishment and growth

Many research studies have shown that spiritual nourishment and growth help people to manage stress better, recover sooner after diseases or operations and generally remain healthier and happier.

Realise that your strength and power lie in your own immortal soul. Listen to your heart and become aware of your inner being.

Spirituality is the universal connection between the mind and the soul. It is a basic human attribute directly from the Creator to all people, no matter what their religion.

12 Communing with nature

We all know instinctively that by getting out and enjoying nature, we are nourishing our bodies and souls. Nature helps us to get our lives back into balance, to realise where we fit in the scheme of things and to appreciate and enjoy life.

Walk in a forest, a park or in your neighbourhood. Look at the animals, the birds and the plants. Be aware of the here and now. Appreciate the small things you overlook every day or take for granted.

3 Health in perspective

No single factor is responsible for health or sickness. Think of the human being as a four level entity comprising body, mind, emotions and soul. Chronic or continual acute diseases in the body such as infections and asthma attacks are almost always a manifestation of a disease in the soul, mind or emotions.

Wellbeing is more than just an absence of the symptoms of disease. It is an inner peace, happiness and joy. It is usually associated with a deep contentment and certainty of your purpose on earth and the conviction that while the body is only temporary, the soul lasts forever.

It is no good treating the symptoms of the body's disease processes without treating the deep-seated sickness in the soul. Even if you don't have a thorough knowledge of psychology (it should be rather be called the study of personality these days!), simply being aware of the close link between body, emotions, mind and soul puts us in a better position to be able to heal ourselves from within. It teaches us to investigate more closely the true origin of our disease.

It is particularly important to realise that children also suffer from stress-related diseases. We are deceiving ourselves if we think of childhood as a dreamy idyllic state of fun-filled carefree days surrounded by the protective love of friends and family. Throughout the world children are increasingly exposed to violence, terror and family rows. The television and news media make children more aware of the ills of a society where almost the only events that are newsworthy are negative. Children are increasingly pressured to achieve more and do better. The technology associated with information overload may sometimes be too much for adults to handle; think of how much more it can affect children.

We must be aware of these factors so that we are on the lookout for deeper-seated psychological problems in children of all ages – especially when they keep getting infections, suffer from allergies and hyperactivity or show antisocial behaviour and signs of depression.

Children are often not able to verbalise their feelings. They bottle them up inside and they are manifested in various symptoms of disease.

The holistic approach to balance and health

The American Holistic Medical Association describes holistic medicine as a system of medical care that emphasises personal involvement. It also encourages a co-operative relationship between all parties involved. It encompasses all safe modalities for diagnosis and treatment while taking account of the whole (holistic means whole) person: physically, emotionally, spiritually and intellectually. Environmental, nutritional and lifestyle factors also play a role.

Diagram 3.1 is a holistic representation of single factors that play a role in the health and balance of the body-mind-emotion-soul entity.

The various factors in the diagram are discussed in random order.

1 Influence of television, music and books

Television can have a positive or negative influence. If you plonk yourself down in front of the television every evening and sit there until bedtime, the television has definitely assumed too much importance in your life. It has become a mindless activity that does not contribute at all to your spiritual growth. Do you feel happy and peaceful after watching the news or a violent programme or film? Such programmes make you sleep badly and you often wake up in the morning feeling tired. An informative, educational programme makes you feel much better. If the news depresses you, don't watch it every night. We only see the bad news and it is often a misrepresentation of what is happening in real life. Good news is seldom 'news'. Choose the programmes you watch with care and encourage your children to watch programmes and films that will enrich them.

Enriching programmes need not only be about fairies and butterflies. There are programmes that illustrate the negative aspects of the personality, where people experience pain and heartache or do terrible things to their fellow beings, but where inner strength and a growth process prevails. One should always be left with the deep insight that we are all free to choose how to handle a situation, with bitterness and hate or with wisdom, love, compassion and inner growth.

Appreciation of music, or simply listening to soothing music, is one of the best ways to relax and become aware of your inner being. Choose music that makes you feel good and happy.

In the same way books can either teach you something or make you feel that you are drowning in a sea of ignorance. If a book is boring or

Diagram 3.1: Mindmap of the holistic approach to homeostasis (internal balance, wellbeing, and health for body and soul)

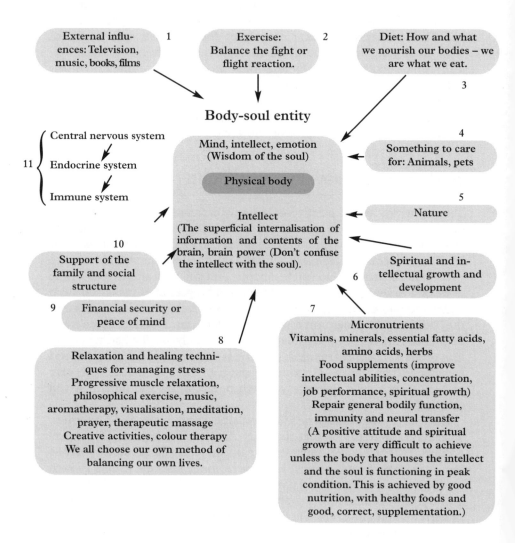

External influences: Television, music, books, films   1

Exercise: Balance the fight or flight reaction.   2

Diet: How and what we nourish our bodies – we are what we eat.

3

Body-soul entity

4

Something to care for: Animals, pets

11
- Central nervous system
- Endocrine system
- Immune system

Mind, intellect, emotion (Wisdom of the soul)

Physical body

5

Nature

Intellect (The superficial internalisation of information and contents of the brain, brain power (Don't confuse the intellect with the soul).

10
Support of the family and social structure

6
Spiritual and intellectual growth and development

9   Financial security or peace of mind

7

8

Relaxation and healing techniques for managing stress
Progressive muscle relaxation, philosophical exercise, music, aromatherapy, visualisation, meditation, prayer, therapeutic massage
Creative activities, colour therapy
We all choose our own method of balancing our own lives.

Micronutrients
Vitamins, minerals, essential fatty acids, amino acids, herbs
Food supplements (improve intellectual abilities, concentration, job performance, spiritual growth)
Repair general bodily function, immunity and neural transfer
(A positive attitude and spiritual growth are very difficult to achieve unless the body that houses the intellect and the soul is functioning in peak condition. This is achieved by good nutrition, with healthy foods and good, correct, supplementation.)

depresses you, leave it. Rely on your intuition or inner guide when it comes to selecting books.

2 Exercise as a physical release for the fight or flight reaction

Exercise gives us the physical outlet our physiology needs to balance the stress reaction. It helps us to move the focus away from our thoughts and concentrate on the here and now. Few things have such a positive, immediate, effect on our body and soul as exercise.

The type of exercise involved here is moderate, pleasurable, regular exercise. Choose something that you enjoy and that you will be able to keep up. Walking is an excellent all-embracing exercise that everyone can fit into a busy schedule. Make time for exercise and enjoy it.

3 Effect of diet on body and soul (how and what we eat to feed our bodies)

Diet in this sense in no way implies any form of deprivation or abstinence from any types or groups of food. If we always eat with the thought 'We become what we eat' in our minds, we usually eat the right kinds of food intuitively. It is not the wrong things that we eat now and then that cause the damage to our minds and bodies, but the wrong things we eat habitually every day.

All macronutrients (proteins, starches and fats) are broken down in the digestive tract into base nutrients: proteins into amino acids, starches (carbohydrates) into glucose, and fats (lipids) into fatty acids and glycerol. The base nutrients are absorbed from the digestive tract and transported by the blood to the liver where they form part of many metabolic processes. Then the nutrients are transported by the blood to all the cells in the body where they are taken up and form part of the thousands of metabolic and biochemical processes that take place every millisecond in every cell day and night. Ultimately, everything that we consume by mouth becomes part of our nuclear matter and the DNA molecules which are responsible for our genetic identity and all cell and organ functions.

If we think of these things while we are eating, we will taste and smell every mouthful and know whether or not we want it to form part of who we are. We will never again have to go on a kilojoule-restricted or crippling diet. We will think of food as the energy source that it should be and give up our daily battle with food. We will make peace with our body's daily needs and no longer use food, especially snack food, as a comfort and replacement for personality defects and emotional gaps.

4 Need to care for someone or something

Frail elderly people in old-age homes were the subjects of a research project. Each resident was given a pet, usually a bird in a cage, to look after. Their general state of health, wellbeing and joie de vivre increased remarkably. Even those who themselves no longer felt like eating or did not originally want to be part of the project found a new interest in life. They once again had something that depended on their care. They had a new goal and purpose in life.

Looking after or taking care of something is a very real human need. We can all care for something or someone. Don't take on more than you can manage – you needn't save the human race. Find something that suits your needs and that you can accommodate into your lifestyle.

5 Communing with nature to ensure balance between body and soul

It is important for all of us to get out into the open and enjoy nature. It helps us to see things in perspective and appreciate the moment.

If you feel that your situation and circumstances are getting too much for you, go for a walk, climb a little hill and look down at the world below. Lift yourself above your circumstances in your imagination. This helps you to view your problem objectively – almost as an observer. You will often find answers and solutions in this way.

It is also good for adults to observe nature in the same way as they did when they were children. Enjoy every moment and marvel at every little thing you see as if you are seeing it for the first time.

6 Awareness of ourselves as spiritual beings with emotional, physical and personal identity

Just as we take care of our bodies to ensure optimal physical functioning, we need to take care of our minds, emotions and souls for its psychic needs.

Read informative books, join groups that will broaden your horizons and exchange your tunnel vision for a new outlook on new spiritual experiences. In our ignorance and fear we often tend to shun strange concepts and new schools of thought. Read about these things and think them over. Take what is good from all religions, philosophies and cultures so that you can extend your mind, soul, intellect and grow.

Awareness of the inner soul helps us to determine what our purpose is on earth and how to apply our talents for the good of the community.

Every person who develops spiritually helps to strengthen and develop the universal consciousness.

7 Micronutrients in the form of vitamins, minerals, essential fatty acids, amino acids and herbs for holistic health

The main part of this book concentrates on the different ways in which micronutrients can restore the function in the different systems of the body-mind unit.

It is difficult to have a positive attitude and grow spiritually if the body, the temporal home of the soul, is not functioning optimally. This is one of the reasons that most peoples' good resolutions often come to nothing. Even if the spirit is willing, but the flesh is weak, it is to the long-term detriment of both.

8 Daily relaxation techniques

Each one of us should set aside time every day for relaxation. Ten minutes morning and evening is enough, but 20 minutes twice a day is even better. This is important for the physiological balance of the stress reaction. If the tension of the day is not restored to balance with some form of relaxation technique, it will eventually take its toll.

There are many relaxation techniques and alternative healing options to try. It is a case of finding the one you feel comfortable with and can identify with. Don't condemn some of the techniques because they don't suit you. Other people may find them very effective. You may not approve of them or want to adopt them, but don't treat other people's choices with suspicion and prejudice.

Chapter 2 deals with the relaxation reaction as a technique for managing stress. Many groups and books offer guidance on meditation, visualisation and practical philosophy. Prayer and a quiet time also give the body and soul time to recover their balance, contemplate the events of the day and then move on. Any form of creative activity and exercise helps the body and mind to relax.

There are many books on colour therapy. It is good to become aware of the role that colour plays in our lives. Don't paint the place where you relax in bright colours such as red, dazzling yellow or orange if you want to relax completely. These are stimulating colours. A light pink is healing and green is the best colour for effective therapy. Blue and green are both calming colours – and by extension turquoise and violet (indigo).

9 Financial security for peace of mind (an abundance of riches)

How can people not worry when they don't know if they'll have enough money to survive? (Obviously we all need enough money to live on.) However, we must see our materialistic drive for external power and money for what it is: a search for inner peace and happiness.

Are you setting your sights too high? Scale down and cut out unnecessary status symbols and expenses. Do the kind of work you enjoy doing. This will immediately shift the emphasis from a regular salary cheque to a more positive attitude. You will begin to think in a spiritual pattern of abundance rather than about the fact that you have to scrimp and save to get to the end of the month. The fear of not having enough results in a constant inner dialogue of negative thoughts and attitude, focussed on need, want and lack.

Abundance is a spiritual condition. We often create our own reality – even at an unconscious level. If we start to think more consciously of where we are going and what we really want to do, the material things will follow of their own accord. However, they will no longer be of primary importance and we will also apply them to the benefit of society. We must learn to convert our dream world into one of abundance, positive actions and wealth. The results will amaze you. Just as with any new pattern of behaviour, it takes time to adopt a positive pattern of thinking. Be patient. Don't reproach yourself if you do not get it right at once.

10 Support in a close family sense and in a broader social context

Children and parents are an essential part of each other's lives. The members of the family must learn from one another, support each other and grow together.

Human beings are social by nature. Our need for contact with our fellow beings is as important as our need for food, water and oxygen.

Research has shown that the people who have a good social support network, recover sooner after a heart attack and are able to get on with their lives much sooner after a bereavement. An example is the support structures that operate in church congregations.

11 Close interaction between the nervous system, endocrine system and immune system

We experience our environment through all our senses. We generate thoughts in our minds. Messages are then sent by the neurotransmitters and hormones throughout our bodies so that every cell and its nucleus can 'feel' and function according to the way the person is feeling.

The white blood cells which are responsible for our resistance to viruses, bacteria and cancer cells contain receptors for the same neurotransmitters that send messages from one nerve ending to another in the nervous system.

If we are continually angry, scared, dissatisfied, unhappy and frustrated, our immune system continually receives negative messages. These do little to encourage the white blood cells to do a proper job of defence!

Be aware of this close interaction and the role your attitude plays in your general health and wellbeing.

Many books have been written on the contribution we make unconsciously to our disease processes (consult the references at the back of the book). Rather than feeling guilty about this, think of how empowering it is to be able to consciously take control of your thoughts, state of mind and ultimately your health.

The best medicine is still preventive medicine. The table on page 40 gives the screening tests that men and women should take at various ages to ensure a long, healthy life. Combine the preventive measures offered by Western technology with lifestyle adjustments and you have a recipe for success.

Table of medical screening tests

Procedure	Men/women/both	Age to start	Frequency	Associated diseases	Comment
History and physical examination with questionnaire on stress	Both	25–40	Every 2 years	Various	Establish knowledge of preventive medicine and body-soul unit awareness at a young age
Homocysteine level (blood test)	Both	20	Every 5 years	Cardiovascular disease	More important than LDL-cholesterol level in determining risk for developing arterial disease
Breast examination	Women	20	Every year	Breast cancer	Include with history and physical examination
Pap smear; vaginal and rectal examination	Women	From onset of sexual activity 14–18	Every 2 years	Cancer of the cervix	
Mammogram	Woman	40–50	Large breasts and family history of breast cancer – every 2 years	Breast cancer	About 14th day of menstrual cycle in premenopausal women (i.e. after start of menstruation)
Full blood count, urea and electrolytes, liver functions, urine analysis, lipid profile, fasting blood sugar	Both	30–40	Every 2 years	Various	Once at 20 years of age in cases of family history and risk factors
Rectal examination	Men	40	Every year	Prostate cancer	Included with history and physical examination
Prostate-specific antigen (PSA) blood tests	Men	40	Every year	Prostate cancer	
Treadmill exertion ECG test	Women Men	50 45	Every year	Cardiovascular	Earlier in cases of risk factors (35 years) such as family history, high cholesterol
Lung function	Both	40	Every year	Respiratory disease	Only for smokers and people with respiratory tract problems

4 Food supplements for optimal health

Supplements are daily additions to a person's normal diet to ensure optimal health and functioning of the body-mind-emotions-spirit unit. They support and strengthen the systems of the body so that the metabolism functions optimally.

Supplements consist mainly of micronutrients such as vitamins, minerals, amino acids, essential fatty acids and medicinal herbs. Macronutrients (macro = big) include carbohydrates (starch), fats and proteins. They are stored in the body and used when needed. Carbohydrates are broken down into glucose to provide energy for all metabolic functions. Fats are broken down into fatty acids and glycerol and stored in the body as fats for conversion into energy. Proteins are broken down into amino acids and then built up in the body into proteins which have many functions in the body. Most of us consume enough macronutrients – or even too many. A balanced diet should always provide sufficient macronutrients. The philosophy, functions and fat phobias surrounding the macronutrients will be discussed in detail in the next book. For the purposes of this book, we will concentrate on the micronutrients.

Micronutrients are nutrients that must be taken daily in small quantities. The American Cancer Association recommends an intake of five to nine portions of fresh fruit and vegetables a day to provide adequate quantities for the daily requirement of micronutrients to prevent cancer and other chronic diseases. (A portion is equal to a large serving spoon or one medium-sized apple, one orange, etc.) Chronic diseases include diabetes, chronic bronchitis and emphysema, arthritis, allergies, chronic fatigue syndrome (yuppy flu or ME), atherosclerosis (thickening of the arteries), high blood pressure, eczema, psoriasis, chronic infections (such as sinusitis) and osteoporosis. Degenerative diseases are those conditions where there is a slow, progressive deterioration in the functioning of a specific system or organ. Diabetes, arthritis and atherosclerosis are examples of degenerative diseases.

The 5-9 a day are the suggested portions intended for the prevention of disease. As soon as we subject the body to an increased workload, our daily need for micronutrients increases accordingly. This happens during the usual stresses of daily life, any form of exercise and also while the body is dealing with a disease process. This sets up a vicious circle: a lack of micronutrients plays an important role in the origin of the disease process. Disease and stress increase the burden on the body, leading it to an increased need for more micronutrients. If these are not provided through diet or food supplements, the disease gets worse and the body's resistance to infectious organisms (viruses, bacteria, fungi and parasites) and stress is reduced.

Eat as many fresh fruit and vegetables a day as possible, but for optimal health also take a good quality food supplement.

Except for freshness, you also need to vary your daily intake of fresh fruit and vegetables. It is no good eating seven apples in one day. Our body requires a wide variety of fruit and vegetables. An example of a balanced intake for a day would include a banana and a large slice of pawpaw for breakfast; a large mixed salad containing lettuce, a tomato, three carrots, an apple, onion and quarter of a cucumber for lunch; and broccoli (lightly cooked), pumpkin (cooked until soft but without butter and sugar!), cauliflower and green beans (both lightly cooked) for supper. Use different kinds of fruit and vegetables every day. Each member in the family will probably have their own interpretation of the words tasty, nutritious and variety!

It is very difficult to comply with this quantity and variety of daily intake of fruit and vegetables. Our lifestyles simply do not permit it. For practical purposes it is therefore essential to take supplementary micronutrients in the form of food supplements. They provide peace of mind and an extra insurance policy, especially for mothers who will be satisfied that the whole family is getting the right micronutrients every day.

The next problem is that we do not always know how fresh the products are when we buy them. Research has shown time and again that the longer fruit and vegetables are removed from their source, the lower their vitamin and mineral content become.

The soil that supplies the nutrients to the plants we eat is often depleted of these nutrients. This can cause marginal deficiencies of a number of micronutrients in the body. (Marginal vitamin status is discussed on page 43.)

Farming methods can also be a problem. Aspects of this include the overfertilisation of soil and excessive use of pesticides, which obviously affect the plants produced in the soil. Fruit and vegetables are often harvested before they are ripe and before they have reached their full nutritional status. The difference in taste between a home-grown tomato and a supermarket tomato reflects the difference in micronutrient values. The methods of crop cultivation often focus on appearance, resistance to insects and transport rather than nutritional value. Fruit such as apples can be kept in cold storage for months until the market needs it. Eventually the product that comes on to the market is quite unlike the original fresh fruit or vegetable – in taste, nutrition value and smell.

Organic farming methods ensure plants with an excellent nutritional status. However, this option is more expensive in the short term; the initial yield is much smaller and there are fewer varieties than commercial farming methods can supply. Ideally all farming industries should change to organic farming methods so that all plants would be of the same excellent quality and size.

Instead of challenging the entire South African farming industry, perhaps we can reach a compromise: use the fresh products available, but supplement their nutritional value with a top-quality food supplement.

Many research studies have proven that food supplements contribute to the prevention of chronic degenerative diseases and should form part of an effective treatment program. Our cells need an abundant supply of micronutrients, including vitamins, minerals, essential fatty acids, amino acids and glucose. To meet this requirement we must follow a healthy, wholesome diet and take the right supplements.

Micronutrients also protect us from environmental toxins and the damage they cause cells. Every day our bodies are bombarded with toxins in food, water, the air, deodorants, cooking utensils, dental fillings, insecticides, etc. Exposure to toxins overloads the detoxification systems in our body. These systems depend on certain vitamins and minerals to function effectively. Deficits in these supporting substances (the micronutrients) eventually lead to health problems. (Antioxidants are discussed in more detail in Chapter 5.)

Marginal vitamin status

The recommended daily allowance (RDA) for micronutrients was worked out many years ago as the minimum daily requirement of vitamins and minerals needed to prevent vitamin-deficiency diseases. Let's take vitamin C as an example. An orange (with good nutritional status) provides about 60 mg of vitamin C. One orange a day is enough to prevent scurvy. (The fresh supply station at the Cape was originally established so that sailors could take fresh products on board.) However, for vitamin C to act as an antioxidant, to treat a disease and boost the immune system, one would need between 1 000 mg and 2 000 mg a day. This is much more than the vitamin C provided by one orange. To meet the body's requirement for vitamin C, we should all take at least 500 mg of vitamin C a day. (Remember, the entire intake need not be in the form of supplements. We also get vitamin C through our diet, but not enough.)

The same principle applies to most vitamins and minerals. By providing our bodies with the minimum recommended daily allowance, we are preventing vitamin-deficiency diseases. But that is not enough. The minimum daily allowance of calcium has been adjusted to achieve optimal nutritional status. The minimum recommended daily allowance (RDA) of calcium has been set at 1 200 mg. To comply with this we must take in at least 600 mg of calcium in an amino acid combination called a chelation. (Calcium and magnesium supplements are discussed in Chapter 10.) Menopausal women should supplement their diet with about 900-1 200 mg of calcium a day (this would include peri-menopausal women who are in the transitional period).

The main functions of vitamins and minerals (as they occur in fresh fruit, vegetables and food supplements) include acting as antioxidants and providing support for the enzymes in the body.

Micronutrients are involved in every biochemical action that takes place in every cell of the body. They act as co-factors (in a co-operative role) or co-enzymes (form part of the enzyme structure) for all the enzymes in the body. Micronutrients also act as hormone regulators and are even involved in the genetic expression of the DNA molecule in each cell nucleus.

Hormones are protein molecules with a very important regulatory effect on all metabolic functions in the body. Hormones are produced in the endocrine glands and then transported to specific target organs via the blood where they have an effect on the functioning of the body. Examples of hormones include insulin and glucagon secreted by the pancreas to control blood sugar, the testosterone from the testes to regulate the male urogenital system and metabolism, the oestrogen and progesterone produced by the ovaries to regulate the female urogenital system and the metabolism, the adrenalin and cortisol secreted by the adrenal glands to regulate the stress reaction, and the thyroid hormones to regulate the metabolic rate of all biochemical reactions.

Enzymes are catalysts which ensure the efficacy, rate and quality of all biochemical reactions in the body. Each cell has thousands of enzymes that contribute to building up (anabolise) or breaking down (catabolise) a wide variety of compounds so that a cell can function effectively.

Let's use water as an example (seeing that our bodies consist of at least 60 per cent water).

$$H \cdot$$
$$H \cdot \quad + \quad \cdot \ddot{O}: \quad \xrightarrow[\text{Enzyme}]{} \quad H : \ddot{O} :$$
$$H$$

$$2 \times H^+ + O$$
(hydrogen)   (oxygen)

H_2O (water)

An enzyme is a complex protein molecule consisting of different amino acid chains. Enzymes are responsible for very specific reactions. The kind, quantity and arrangement of the amino acids determine the type of enzyme.

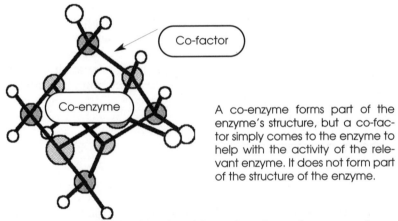

Co-factor

Co-enzyme

A co-enzyme forms part of the enzyme's structure, but a co-factor simply comes to the enzyme to help with the activity of the relevant enzyme. It does not form part of the structure of the enzyme.

If enzymes become depleted or sluggish, or they do not have enough co-enzymes and co-factors, the reactions they are responsible for will also diminish or become sluggish. The functioning of the cells will become sluggish as well. Eventually the organ will become sluggish and the effective functioning of an entire system will be affected. This is exactly what happens at the onset of many diseases of our time. The specific system that is affected depends on genetic susceptibility, and the effect of stress, lifestyle and environment. The weak links in the enzyme chains will be the first to break. The weak link is the genetically transmitted susceptibility inherited from our ancestors that will cause certain diseases in specific systems. (Examples are asthma, high blood pressure, eczema, atherosclerosis and diabetes.)

The main cause of enzyme failure is lack of support by co-enzymes and co-factors which are the vitamins, minerals and other micronutrients.

The immune system is often the first system to suffer as a result of reduced enzyme functioning. In the short term this leads to chronic infections and in the long term it could cause cancer in genetically susceptible individuals.

Marginal vitamin status is a grey area between optimal health and the clinical vitamin-deficiency diseases. There are degrees of deterioration in vitamin status: at first there is simply a decline in the feeling of wellbeing, and later chronic degenerative diseases develop. These deficiencies do not happen overnight – they occur over a long period of time.

Vitamin depletion goes through different stages. At first the tissue storage depots where particular vitamins are stored are diminished. This leads to a weakening of cellular biochemical functioning and non-specific symptoms appear.

Let's use vitamin C as an example again. With a marginal deficiency of vitamin C, weakened immune function will manifest long before any signs of scurvy (vitamin-deficiency disease) are detected. Scurvy will probably never develop, as the individual takes in enough vitamin C to prevent a vitamin-deficiency disease from developing, but the person's metabolism will not function optimally.

Stages of vitamin depletion

The various stages of vitamin depletion can be described as follows:

1 Precursor stage: There is less storage of specific vitamins and minerals in the tissues as a result of a reduced intake of micronutrients, or an abnormal metabolism where high demands are made on the metabolism and thus the enzymes and micronutrients (in cases of diabetes, surgery, severe long-term tension or stress and active participation in sport). Symptoms include increased fatigue, listlessness and vague complaints of a reduced feeling of wellbeing or vitality.

2 Biochemical stage: There is a reduction in enzyme activity and a change in metabolism. This stage can be measured by looking at the end result of a specific enzyme's activity. If it is too low, the conclusion is that the enzyme is not functioning efficiently. These tests are expensive and not very practical.

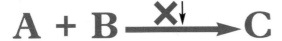

If enzyme X does not appear to be functioning properly, the end product for which X is responsible, namely C, can be measured. If C is low, enzyme X needs boosting.

3 Physiological stage: The enzyme activity is reduced even further. Reduced enzyme concentrations can be measured by determining the concentration of a specific enzyme in the blood. Symptoms relating to this stage include loss of appetite, severe fatigue, listlessness, depression and disturbed sleep, reduced immune function with continual niggling infections. Most chronic diseases would fall in this category.

4 Clinical stage: The non-specific symptoms are aggravated and the classic symptoms and signs of the vitamin-deficiency diseases (rickets, pellagra, beri-beri or scurvy) appear. Patients improve dramatically if given the correct vitamins, mainly through injections. This proves just how important micronutrients are for good health.

5 Anatomical stage: The changes and degeneration in tissue morphology are so far advanced that, unless there is timeous intervention using the correct vitamin therapy, the patient will die.

Only stages 4 and 5 have clear clinical symptoms. Most people never deteriorate as far as these two stages, because the minimal daily intake of micronutrients will prevent it.

The first three stages of actual marginal deficiencies will often not manifest until the body is subjected to increased stress or a greater burden such as surgery, tension at work, disease, allergies, a marathon, injury or increased stress and tension.

A person in stage 1 who is suddenly subjected to surgery will deteriorate to stages 2 or 3 as a result of the additional demands made on the body's enzymes. After surgery the immune system is very sensitive and the liver has to break down the anaesthetic drugs with the aid of effective enzyme action into harmless waste material which can be excreted by the kidneys or bowel. The sensitivity of the immune system and increased liver enzyme activity result in slower postoperative recovery and infections can set in. A person whose vitamin status is optimal will have few postoperative side effects. Recovery will be quick, with minimal formation of scar tissue and very few side effects from the anaesthetic drugs. The person will be able to return to work soon after the operation, feeling fine.

Any disease process can follow the same course. As soon as vitamin and mineral supplements are taken, the body systematically returns through all the stages back to optimal health. This is why people who regularly take good supplements eventually find that their symptoms and disease will improve. But be patient; it takes time. The deficiency first has to be restored at tissue level so that enzyme activity can improve. The longer the existence of the disease process, the longer it takes to return to good health back along the same gradient as the deterioration took place.

If you choose the right dosage of the right supplements, and adopt healthy eating habits, regular exercise, lifestyle adjustment and stress management, you can return step by step (from stage 4, to stage 3, to stage 2 and to stage 1) to a state of optimum health and wellbeing. It is never too late to use supplements. Of course, it is advisable to start with corrective action sooner rather than later, but any person can take control of their own health at any time. Even a person in the advanced stages of cancer will experience an improved quality of life, and less fatigue, loss of appetite and nausea. Remember that micronutrients are an inextricable part of our neurotransmitters, hormonal and immune system. They play a major role in determining our state of mind and the development of inner wisdom. If you do not have enough micronutrients for your daily needs, you are unable to function optimally either mentally, emotionally or physically. (Antioxidants are discussed in chapter 5 and supporting the nervous system in Chapter 12.)

Choosing the right supplements

By now you should be convinced and aware of the need to take food supplements. They are a good preventive measure and an excellent health insurance policy. Your next question would probably be which combinations you need and how much to take.

The rest of this book deals with the specific needs of certain people and in certain systems of the body where genetically weakened enzyme activity manifests itself in disease processes. These are general guidelines to give guidance and take the guesswork out of choosing the right supplements.

Individual needs may differ greatly according to the genetic determination of enzyme activity. If some people have inherited a sensitive or weak enzyme activity in specific organs or systems, they may require more than others. The role of heredity is important only if the individual's capacity to manage stress and attitude to life tend to be negative and their general lifestyle is below par (because of poor dietary habits, unhealthy food, lack of exercise, smoking, too much alcohol, etc.).

The recommended doses for supplements in this chapter and in the following chapters are indicated as a general guideline for the specific system. Some people may need more; others less. These are not prescriptive quantities, but merely an aid and guideline to simplify your choices. If you have a disease in one of the systems, you will need more. If you only want to prevent disease or want to be healthier, you will need less.

Remember that combination and synergy (co-operation) of vitamins, minerals and other micronutrients are more important than the quantities of single micronutrients. If the quantity is less than that recommended in this book, but the supplement contains a number of other micronutrients, you can use less of each ingredient. Always take vitamins and minerals with meals for better absorption, especially the fat-soluble ones (vitamins A, D and E). Always take calcium and magnesium at night to ensure a better night's sleep. Vitamin C should be divided into two or three doses and taken throughout the day to ensure constant blood levels.

Calcium is the only supplement where a minimum daily allowance of 600 mg of absorbable calcium (in a good chelation), combined with a minimum of 300 mg of magnesium is strongly recommended.

Three basic products are required. Unfortunately, the right quantities of each are not obtainable in one single supplement. If they were, it would be the size of a saucer!

1. We should all take a **calcium and magnesium supplement** (600 mg of calcium and 300 mg of magnesium for teenagers and adults and 900-1 200 mg of calcium and 450-600 mg of magnesium for women over 50 at night). The supplement should also contain vitamins D and C. (The role of calcium and magnesium is discussed in Chapter 10.)

2. We should take a supplement of **essential fatty acids** in the form of omega-3 (for example, 250-1 000 mg of salmon oil or EPA) and omega-6 fatty acids (for example 500-1 000 mg of evening primrose oil or GLA) every day. (Essential fatty acids are discussed in Chapter 9.)

3. We should take a good **multivitamin and antioxidant combination** every day. (If you have problems with a specific system in the body, refer to the chapter on that system for the suitable combinations and quantities.) Remember, we are not neatly divided into systems! The method of presentation is merely for practical purposes and because diseases manifest in certain systems on account of genetic susceptibility and stress.

If no specific system is affected, you can take a general multivitamin and antioxidant combination that complies with the following requirements:

- Know yourself and your body's needs. We all know instinctively if something is lacking in our minds or bodies. Discuss your needs with your health care provider. Find someone who is knowledgeable about micronutrients. Many doctors and health care providers scoff at the idea of supplements or say they are unnecessary. This indicates a shocking lack of knowledge that is freely available today. Thousands of research articles, books and Internet publications can be found that prove the need to take supplements. You can also easily extend your own knowledge on the subject.
- Supplements made of natural plant extracts and products are better absorbed and utilised by the body. Although laboratory tests show that synthetic supplements are just as easily absorbed, the body can distinguish between natural and synthetic nutrients. The body recognises and absorbs natural plant extracts more efficiently. Always take your supplements with meals, usually with breakfast and supper. Micronutrients are taken naturally with food, digested and absorbed. This also reminds you to take the supplements regularly. It is no good taking supplements every now and then. Be patient before you expect results. It can take four weeks to three months before there is a marked improvement in your general health.
- It is preferable to take minerals in a chelated form to ensure optimal absorption from the intestines, optimal bioavailability to the cells where they must function, as well as optimal biological activity or performance. This means that minerals should be bound to amino acids in a chelation. This is the best way to ensure that all the micronutrients you take reach the cells. Amino acids are the building blocks of proteins and also a natural part of the body. By taking minerals in this form, you can take less and the possibility of side effects such as bloating, black stools, nausea and constipation caused by poor compounds is reduced. Make sure that your minerals are in an

amino acid chelation.

- Micronutrients work together synergistically in complex ways. It is recommended that you take a micronutrient combination rather than one, two or three micronutrients on their own. Research has shown that combinations of micronutrients can alleviate almost any health problem. Take heart problems, for instance. Vitamin E is very important for the recovery of heart muscle function after a heart attack and for preventing atherosclerosis, but vitamins C and A, the minerals selenium, zinc and magnesium, the B-complex vitamins, the essential fatty acids, the amino acid carnitine and the co-enzyme Q10 are also essential for the optimal functioning and recovery of the heart. So do not use vitamin E on its own.

- Your choice should include the following (quantities given are the total daily dosage):

Vitamin A with 60 per cent in the form of beta and mixed carotenes: about 5 000 international units (IU) or 1 500 micrograms (1,5 mg) of vitamin A and a minimum of 25 000 IU (15 mg) of beta carotene and mixed carotenes or carotenoids.

Vitamin C: Your multivitamin complex should contain about 250 mg of vitamin C. The total daily supplement for vitamin C is about 500 mg. If the multivitamin contains too little vitamin C, remember that your calcium supplement should also contain vitamin C. In any event it is advisable to take vitamin C more than once a day. (Take calcium and magnesium in the evenings at bedtime. So you have vitamin C in the morning with your multivitamin and in the evening with your calcium and magnesium.)

Vitamin E, 100-200 IU (or 83-166 mg) a day, preferably in all four forms of vitamin E (alpha, beta, delta and gamma) also in the natural d form (such as d-alpha tocopherol).

Vitamin B-complex, about 25 mg of each (B1, B2, B3, B5, B6 occur mainly as a group). Remember that folic acid is also a B vitamin (200 micrograms a day). Vitamin B12 is usually taken in a quantity of about 25-50 micrograms a day. Choline, lecithin, inositol, para amino benzoic acid (PABA), 25 mg of each a day and biotin (25 micrograms a day) are also included in the B-complex vitamins.

Minerals (preferably in amino acid chelation)

Selenium, 100 micrograms (take all components together), Chromium 200 micrograms, Zinc 15 mg, Copper 2 mg, Iron 15 mg (for premenopausal, pregnant and breastfeeding women only), Manganese 10 mg.

The above quantities are for a person of average health who wants to remain healthy. In the case of disease, greater dosages are required.

Phytonutrients (plant nutrients) such as the bioflavonoids quercetin, green tea, acerola cherry extract, tomato powder with lycopene, broccoli powder extract with sulphoraphane, grape seed extract with proanthocyanidin, alfalfa (lucerne) extract with lutein are some examples. Any phytonutrients in your multivitamin combination is beneficial to your health.

The combination can also contain the following (not essential): the amino acids L-carnitine, lysine, proline, L-glutamine, taurine and glycine, co-enzyme Q10 and the potent antioxidant glutathione (1 mg).

4. Do not forget herbs! Herbs are plants with healing, aromatic and culinary properties. Most herbs have all three characteristics. When you add herbs to your food, you are not only improving the taste and aroma of the dish, you are benefitting from the healing properties of the herbs. Only a few general examples are mentioned here. More herbs are discussed where they are applicable in the sections on the different systems of the body.

Garlic, ginger, turmeric, thyme, rosemary, basil and sage are herbs with a wealth of healing properties – they also improve the taste, flavour and texture of most foods. Grow your own herbs and use them generously in food or take them as a tea.

Essential oils of lavender, camomile, neroli and sandalwood can be added to a bath to relieve stress and anxiety. These herbs can also be taken as a tea.

Echinacea, garlic, nasturtium leaves, camomile, sage and thyme are natural antibiotics which also boost the immune system. (Read more about natural alternatives to antibiotics in Chapter 13.)

5. Amino acids are the building blocks of proteins. Many people either cannot metabolise amino acids in sufficient quantities or have existing enzyme deficiencies. Amino acid deficiencies are a common feature of

our lives today. Amino acid supplements can be valuable for many disease processes in the body. Some of the most important amino acids available in local food supplements are discussed in the relevant chapters where they play a role. It is seldom necessary to take more than one or two amino acid supplements.

Unlike other micronutrients, amino acids must be taken in the morning on an empty stomach with a little fruit juice, vitamin C (250 mg) and B6 (100 mg) for optimal absorption and bioavailability.

Can too many vitamins be dangerous?

Remember, if a little of something is good for you, it does not necessarily mean that more is better.

The toxicity of vitamins is often a topic for debate. People are so concerned about vitamin poisoning, yet they don't bother to read the package inserts of their ordinary prescription medicines or even insist that they be included with the medicine. The package inserts contain a long list of the specific medicine's side effects. Read these and then decide on the actual benefit of the medication. Discuss the side effects with your doctor. Remember that medicine is often prescribed to treat symptoms which are actually the side effects of other medicines.

Vitamins are divided into fat-soluble and water-soluble vitamins. Fat-soluble vitamins include vitamins A, E, D and K. The water-soluble vitamins are the B-complex vitamins, carotenes and vitamin C. The fat-soluble vitamins are stored in the body, while the water-soluble ones are easily excreted. The water-soluble vitamins seldom cause toxicity, especially if you follow the recommended guidelines.

The recent vitamin C scare

A British study, published in the magazine *Nature* (9 April 1998) and in the *New York Times*, alleged that, although vitamin C is an effective antioxidant, it should only be taken in dosages of less than 60 mg a day. Dosages of above 500 mg apparently caused cell damage in research subjects. The study was done with 30 volunteers who took 500 mg of vitamin C daily over a period of six weeks. Before and after the intake of the vitamin, researchers monitored two indicators for oxidative damage in the DNA molecule. The one indicator showed a reduction in oxidation during the vitamin intake, while the other indicator showed more oxidation after than before taking the vitamin. This contradictory and confusing article caused an outcry.

Professor Balz Frei, director of the Linus Pauling Institute, said the findings contradicted other research. The investigation also focussed on a single biological indicator which had not been irrefutably proven to be a good indicator of oxidative stress and cell damage. The well-researched and proven value of vitamin C in risk reduction in cancer, cardiovascular disorders and other serious health problems should be weighed against a single, flawed study that focussed on one aspect of a biological effect.

According to Alex G. Schauss, PhD, director of the Life Science Department of Research on Natural and Medicinal Products, the study did not report that vitamin C caused clinical damage. The researchers found that vitamin C worked as an antioxidant by neutralising the oxygen atoms of certain free radicals, thereby suppressing the growth of cancer. Vitamin C supplementation is therefore quite justified.

In the absence of any more authoritative information which irrefutably proves the opposite, my family and I will continue to use at least 1 000 mg of vitamin C every day in doses of 500 mg in the morning and 500 mg in the evening.

Fat-soluble vitamins

Fat-soluble vitamins may cause toxicity, but this is very rare.

Vitamin A may cause chronic toxicity only with a daily intake in excess of 50 000 IU (15 000 micrograms or 15 mg of retinol equivalent or RE per day). This far exceeds the amounts found in supplements. Symptoms of toxicity include increased pressure in the cerebrospinal fluid (in the brain and spinal cord), dermatitis and liver damage. The symptoms can usually be reversed if the high dosages are stopped.

If the water-soluble precursor beta carotene (or mixed carotenes) is taken as a main source of vitamin A, toxicity will never occur. The body converts the carotene into vitamin A as and when needed.

Children under the age of four should not take more than 5 000 IU of pure vitamin A a day (1 500 micrograms or 1,5 mg of RE). Children older than four and adults do not need more than 10 000 IU (3 000 micrograms or 3 mg of RE) a day. Pregnant women and women who are breastfeeding should not take more than 8 000 IU (2 400 micrograms or 2,4 mg of RE) a day.

Vitamin D can be very potent and therefore toxic, but only with an intake in excess of 25 000 IU a day for adults. Most supplements contain the recommended daily allowance (RDA) of 400-800 IU. Toxicity is therefore extremely rare.

Vitamin E seldom causes toxicity, even when massive daily doses are taken.

Vitamin K, essential for blood clotting, is seldom included in supplements. The natural bacteria in our intestines manufacture enough vitamin K for our requirements. It is only prescribed for people after large sections of their intestine have been removed.

In conclusion

Micronutrients restore the functions of the body. They are not miracle cures. They simply help the body-mind unit to perform all its functions effectively so that you can thrive in a condition of optimal health and wellbeing.

Use your supplements regularly and in the correct quantities and combinations. Eat healthy, wholesome food. Use alcohol sparingly or not at all. Do not smoke. Practise stress management techniques for physical, emotional, spiritual and mental health. Adopt a positive attitude to life. Laugh a lot. Do regular, moderate exercise. You will have an excellent chance of living to a ripe, healthy, wise and fit age of 120 years!

5 Antioxidants

An antioxidant is exactly what is says: against oxygen. Every living thing needs oxygen. But certain kinds of oxygen can be dangerous and detrimental to our health.

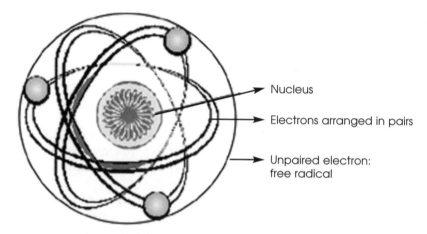

Nucleus

Electrons arranged in pairs

Unpaired electron:
free radical

Schematic representation of an atom with its nucleus and electrons arranged in three pairs around the nucleus. The unpaired electron moving on the outer perimeter is the free radical.

During all the metabolic processes in the body, abnormal oxygen is constantly formed. In a normal oxygen atom two pairs of electrons revolve around the nucleus. This is how the oxygen atom remains in balance. During the metabolic processes in the body, oxygen (*and* hydrogen) atoms acquire an extra unpaired electron. This makes the oxygen atom unstable and biochemically very active. Oxygen or hydrogen atoms such as these are called free radicals. They want to pass the extra electron on to the nearest neighbour (or remove an electron from the nearest neighbour) so that a paired group of electrons again revolves in the outer ring of the atom. The atom will go to any length to recover a natural balance or equilibrium. However, the process turns the neighbour into a free radical. This sets up a vicious circle and a chain reaction is set in motion that can cause extensive cell damage.

This reaction of free radical formation can occur in the cell membrane, which eventually causes the membrane with its phospholipid chains to break. This leads to a leaking of the content of the cell and the cell loses its function. Free radicals can also damage the cell nucleus, where the sensitive DNA molecule which controls all cell functions is found. Free radicals can destroy enzyme systems and damage mitochondria (the energy centres of every cell where all the energy for the cell's requirements is generated).

Formation of free radicals

Free radicals are mainly formed in four ways:
- Free radicals are formed during the generation of energy in the cell – they are the by-products of the electron transfer metabolic chain.
- The detoxification and neutralising of foreign substances such as medication, alcohol, toxins and chemicals which generate large numbers of free radicals.
- When the immune system is activated to eliminate or neutralise foreign organisms (bacteria, parasites and fungi), abnormal cells (such as cancer cells) and foreign protein molecules, the white blood cells produce free radicals to attack these invaders. After the attack, however, the increased number of free radicals remain in the cells and blood.
- Free radicals can enter the body from outside such as ultraviolet light, air pollution and pesticides, as well as from inside such as poor diet and medication.

Examples of free radicals are the superoxide radical, hydrogen peroxide radical, singlet oxygen radical and hydroxyl radical.

Free radicals are extremely destructive and can cause irreparable damage to the delicate biochemical harmony and balance between the cell and the nucleus.

If the DNA growth control centre is damaged, cells can lose the ability to know when they should stop dividing and growing. Cells can also lose their ability to differentiate and they will no longer remember what kind of cell they are. The DNA of every cell contains the memory of the function of every other cell in the body. If the codes become confused, a liver cell could suddenly start growing uncontrollably and develop into a muscle cell where there should not be any muscle cells. This is what

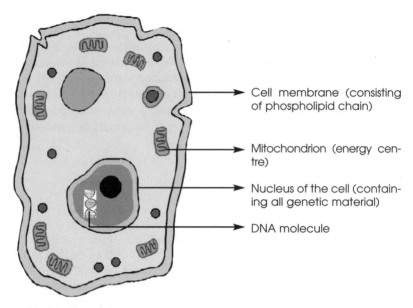

Cell membrane (consisting of phospholipid chain)

Mitochondrion (energy centre)

Nucleus of the cell (containing all genetic material)

DNA molecule

A typical cell in the body

happens in many types of cancer. Cells grow uncontrollably and without differentiation in a suicidal frenzy. The cancer cells eventually destroy the total functioning of an organ, even destroying themselves in the process.

The good news is that there are three antioxidant enzymes in every cell to keep these free radicals under control. They are superoxide dismutase, catalase and glutathione peroxidase. These enzymes donate an electron to the hyperactive oxygen and hydrogen radicals, which are then neutralised and rendered harmless. However, these enzymes cannot always cope with all the free radicals that are formed for the following reasons:

1 Increased production of free radicals (more free radicals are produced than the three enzymes can handle):

● This often happens to people who participate in sports competitively – the more active and competitive they are, the more free radicals are formed on account of the increased metabolism. Active sportsmen and women should therefore take antioxidant supplements to cope with the increased production of free radicals in their bodies. This would improve their performance and increase their endurance – the damage caused by free radicals is reduced and the immune system is boosted, which means fewer infections.

- People who suffer from diabetes have an abnormal glucose metabolism combined with oxidative stress (which increases oxidation – thereby increasing the production of free radicals). Supplementary antioxidants restrict the tissue damage associated with diabetes, reduce the need for insulin and limit the eventual damage to the end organs (kidney damage, nerve damage, eye damage and gangrene) so often linked with the disease. Diabetes is discussed in greater detail at the end of this chapter.

- All forms of chronic disease (such as arthritis, chronic fatigue, chronic infections, emphysema, multiple sclerosis, Alzheimer's disease, atherosclerosis, high cholesterol, varicose veins, cancer and AIDS) results in an increased production of free radicals, which spreads the damage caused by the disease and aggravates and prolongs the disease process.

- Prolonged or uncontrolled stress over a long period can significantly increase the metabolism. The enzymes responsible for maintaining the stress metabolism work harder and the free radicals increase significantly. The body therefore requires support from supplementary antioxidants.

2 Increased exposure to free radicals from the environment is another possibility:

- Smoke – cigarette smoke (inhaled directly or indirectly) and industrial smoke from factories and fires.
- Air pollution caused by factories, vehicle exhaust fumes and heaters.
- Exposure to ultraviolet light, including excessive exposure to sunlight.
- In genetically susceptible people, exposure to carcinogens (substances that cause cancer).

3 The ageing process exerts increasing demands on the enzymes and the enzymes also become less active. Ageing is the sum total of the damage caused by free radicals over a lifetime. It is never too late to take antioxidant supplements, but if you wish to slow down the ageing process the sooner the better. Remember that mental attitude and general lifestyle also play a major role in the ageing process.

4 The immune system is an extremely active system. The enzymes work at top speed to protect you against pollution, carcinogens, viruses, bacteria, fungi and every foreign invader imaginable. The lifestyle we lead today puts a high demand on the immune system. Unless we take antioxidants to boost the immune system, we will suffer the consequences. The white blood cells also produce free radicals to destroy foreign invaders. The free radicals are then released into the surrounding tissue and may aggravate tissue damage. Antioxidants help to prevent and control this process.

The antioxidants we take in through our normal daily diet cannot supply all our needs. The main antioxidant nutrients are beta carotene (and the other carotenes), vitamins A, E and C and the minerals selenium, zinc, copper and manganese. Examples of antioxidants are pycnogenol (found in pine bark and grape seed extract), the co-enzyme Q10 (essential in the mitochondria or power generators of our cells), cat's claw, alpha lipoic acid and glutathione.

All fresh fruit and vegetables are excellent sources of antioxidants. It is, however, virtually impossible to supply all our body's daily needs through diet alone.

> Damage caused by free radicals plays a role in
> almost every modern disease.
> Everyone will benefit from taking antioxidants.

Functions of antioxidants

1 Antioxidants destroy free radicals. They donate electrons, thereby neutralising the free radicals and limiting the damage. This is a very important function in all chronic degenerative diseases, the treatment of AIDS, the prevention and treatment of cancer, the prevention of ageing and any other condition where there is an increased production of free radicals (such as participating in sports and in diabetes). Some antioxidants such as proanthocyanidin (pycnogenol), found in grape seeds and pine bark, penetrate the blood-brain barrier and restrict the damage caused by free radicals inside the brain. This is especially important in the treatment and prevention of stroke, Alzheimer's disease and other forms of dementia.

2 Antioxidants directly boost the performance of the immune system. They increase the adult white blood cell count and improve the existing functioning of the immune system. They considerably improve the body's inherent ability to defend itself against pathogens. This involves healing and supporting the body's own activity, namely its defence mechanisms. A pathogen is any substance that has the potential to cause disease in the body (bacteria, viruses – including those that cause AIDS, carcinogens, fungi and parasites). Antioxidants alleviate the severity of symptoms associated with various infections and reduce the duration of infections. The frequency of infections also decreases markedly. In autoimmune diseases, where the immune system attacks its own cells, such as in systemic lupus erythematosis (SLE), rheumatoid arthritis, Graves' disease and Crohn's disease, antioxidants will enable the immune system to function more normally.

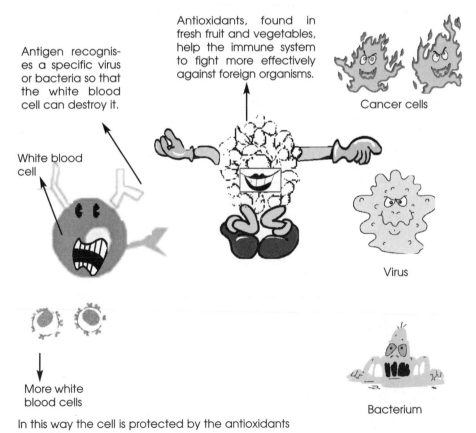

Antigen recognises a specific virus or bacteria so that the white blood cell can destroy it.

Antioxidants, found in fresh fruit and vegetables, help the immune system to fight more effectively against foreign organisms.

Cancer cells

White blood cell

Virus

More white blood cells

Bacterium

In this way the cell is protected by the antioxidants

Antioxidants support the immune system of people who have to undergo chemotherapy or radiotherapy for cancer. The therapy causes a considerable increase in free radical formation and it suppresses immune function as it kills off all fast growing cells (cancer cells grow at an abnormal rate, but the white blood cells, those which cause hair growth and the cells in the digestive tract also grow and divide rapidly).

This is why people who undergo these treatments suffer from so many side effects, including nausea, fatigue and infections. Antioxidants boost the immune system and reduce the other side effects so that the cancer can be fought with a stronger immune system and a more positive mental attitude. Every person who is undergoing any form of cancer treatment should take antioxidant supplements. It is never too late to start. No matter how long you live, you can improve your quality of life. There are no contraindications – in fact, the therapy will be more effective. The notion that folic acid can counteract the effectiveness of the therapy is dated and based on medical opinion of 30 years ago.

3 Antioxidants prevent the oxidation of LDL-cholesterol. (Cholesterol as a lifestyle disease is discussed in Chapter 8.) LDL-cholesterol must be oxidised before it can penetrate the walls of the blood vessels to start the process of atherosclerosis (thickening of the arteries). Antioxidants prevent this oxidation of LDL-cholesterol.

4 Antioxidants form an integral part of the biochemical structure of the body's own antioxidant enzymes. Glutathione peroxidase (GP) increases the concentration of vitamin E thereby improving vitamin E's antioxidant effect. Selenium is an essential co-factor of glutathione peroxidase. Copper, manganese and zinc are part of the structure of superoxide dismutase. Antioxidants maintain and improve the activity and integrity of these essential enzymes.

GP

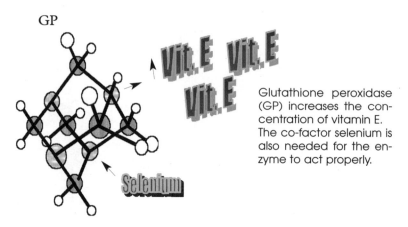

Glutathione peroxidase (GP) increases the concentration of vitamin E. The co-factor selenium is also needed for the enzyme to act properly.

5 Antioxidants suppress and neutralise the effect of carcinogens, so that the triggering process in the development of cancer does not occur. Some antioxidants bind with cell receptors, and prevent the carcinogens from penetrating the cells.

6 Antioxidants have the inherent ability to cause cancer cells to return to normal by restoring the growth control function of cells in the DNA molecule of the cell nucleus. Antioxidants can restore the essential communication between cells. The communication via gap junctions have a restrictive effect on the growth of cancerous cells. Cancer cells lose their ability to communicate with normal cells.

Communication between two normal cells

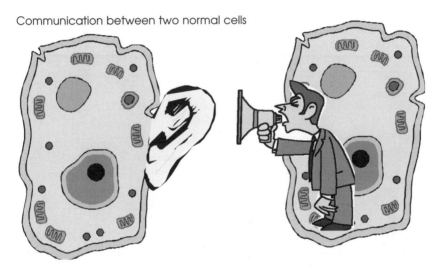

Cells communicate with each other continuously so that function and growth can constantly be monitored. Cancer cells lose this ability which is so essential to life. Antioxidants restore the channels of communication.

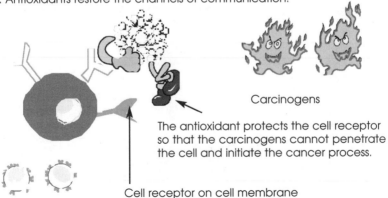

Carcinogens

The antioxidant protects the cell receptor so that the carcinogens cannot penetrate the cell and initiate the cancer process.

Cell receptor on cell membrane

Schematic representation of how the cell is protected by the antioxidants

Diagram 5.1: Stages in the development of cancer and the role of antioxidants

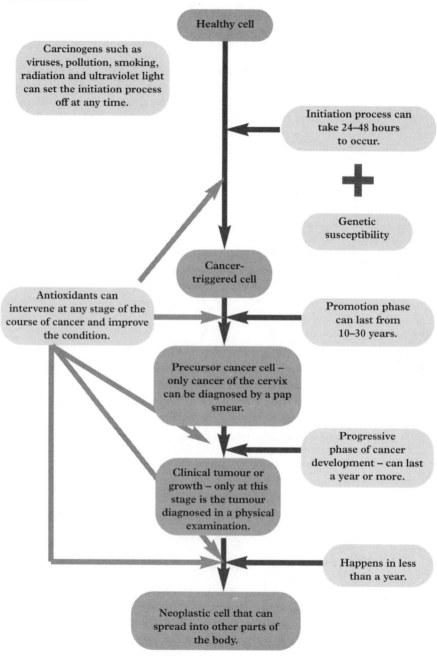

Healthy cell

Carcinogens such as viruses, pollution, smoking, radiation and ultraviolet light can set the initiation process off at any time.

Initiation process can take 24–48 hours to occur.

Genetic susceptibility

Cancer-triggered cell

Antioxidants can intervene at any stage of the course of cancer and improve the condition.

Promotion phase can last from 10–30 years.

Precursor cancer cell – only cancer of the cervix can be diagnosed by a pap smear.

Progressive phase of cancer development – can last a year or more.

Clinical tumour or growth – only at this stage is the tumour diagnosed in a physical examination.

Happens in less than a year.

Neoplastic cell that can spread into other parts of the body.

Antioxidant supplements available in South Africa

*With recommended daily dosages for optimal health

It is important to remember that antioxidants work best in synergy. Each antioxidant has a specific function in the body, but it needs the support of most of the other antioxidants. Antioxidants work in a synchronised way – they never work on their own. Scientists have not yet established all the different ways in which antioxidants work together. They are all linked to one another, work synergistically, depend on each other and are in balance. Ideally, they should be taken in the form of fresh fruit and vegetables. Unfortunately, the percentage of people who consume the recommended five to nine portions of fresh fruit and vegetables a day is estimated at less than 10 per cent of the total population. Try to eat as many fresh fruit and vegetables as possible. Food such as *Rosa roxburghii*, raw honey, certain algae and whole red grapes (skin and pips) contain most of the antioxidants. It is, however, essential for all of us to supplement our diet with a broad spectrum antioxidant formula. People who are suffering from cancer must take twice the recommended dosages.

When choosing antioxidants, the quantity of each individual ingredient is less important than finding a combination that contains as many antioxidants in one product as possible.

If you can divide your daily intake throughout the day, it is better than taking it all at once. This will ensure that levels of antioxidants in the blood remain constant. However, amino acids should be taken on their own on an empty stomach, in conjunction with vitamins C (250 mg) and B6 (50-100 mg). It is unnecessary to take more than one amino acid supplement at a time.

1 Beta and mixed carotenes and vitamin A
(15 000-25 000 IU or 9-15 mg of beta and mixed carotenes and 5 000-10 000 IU of vitamin A for adults a day) (1 microgram of vitamin A activity = 3,3 IU of vitamin A; so 1 500 micrograms or 1,5 mg of retinol equivalent or RE)

Beta and other carotenes act as antioxidants on their own and they are also converted to vitamin A as and when the body needs it. Vitamin A and beta carotene need vitamins C and E for optimal functioning – an example of synergism. There are more than 400 identified carotenoids

– beta carotene is one of them. The supplement you use should contain combinations of different carotenes.

Vitamin A (retinol) is important for night vision. It maintains the structure of the cornea (outer membrane) of the eye and prevents irritation and infection of the eye covering. Vitamin A is often prescribed for the treatment of cataracts, glaucoma, myopia (shortsightedness) and conjunctivitis.

Vitamin A delays the ageing process, especially of the skin, and it can also be applied externally for absorption through the skin. It is strongly recommended for the treatment and management of all stages of acne and other skin complaints such as eczema and psoriasis. Vitamin A also accelerates the recovery of the skin and other tissue after injury and surgery. (Use a vitamin A cream and take a tablet orally.)

Vitamin A reduces the chances of a stroke and limits the brain damage after a stroke. The decreased supply of oxygen, glucose and other nutrients to the area of the brain furthest from the obstruction (the part of the brain distal to the obstruction), causes a considerable accumulation of free radicals. This increases the area of damage in the brain, aggravates the consequences of the stroke and leads to increased nerve fall out. Vitamin A limits this damage.

Vitamin A improves the body's resistance to infections, especially in the respiratory system, urogenital system and alimentary tract. In all these systems it supports the mucosal lining (protective mucous membrane) and ensures a rapid recovery after any infection or inflammation process of the mucous lining.

The carotenes and vitamin A protect the body against the damage of free radicals from smoke and other pollutants. Both play an essential role in the prevention and treatment of almost all types of cancer. They are also very effective in the treatment of ulcers (open sores on the skin or in the mouth) and atherosclerosis where they neutralise free radicals. The carotenes provide protection against cardiovascular disease.

2 Vitamin E and selenium
(100-200 IU or 83-166 mg of vitamin E and 100-200 micrograms of selenium a day)

These two micronutrients work together and are therefore discussed together. It is a good idea to take vitamin E in all four configurations, namely alpha, beta, delta and gamma (for example d-alpha tocopherol). The d configuration is the more natural form of vitamin E (compared to the synthetic dl-configuration). The d-alpha tocopherol configuration of vitamin E is the most potent suppressor of cancer cell growth.

Vitamin C helps vitamin E to recirculate so that it can protect cell membranes from free radicals. Vitamin E prevents vitamin A from being broken down. Vitamin E also prevents fats from becoming rancid in the body. All these functions are examples of synergy.

Vitamin E is often prescribed for premenstrual tension, menstrual irregularities and for the relief of menopausal hot flushes and other menopausal symptoms. It can also be applied externally as a cream to retard the ageing of skin.

Vitamin E and selenium provide protection against cardiovascular disease. It is important to take high dosages especially after a heart attack. In the area beyond the obstruction of the blood vessel there is a considerable accumulation of free radicals in the heart tissue furthest from the obstruction (distal). This results in a more extensive area of tissue damage. Taking vitamin E and selenium after a heart attack accelerates the rate of recovery much quicker and reduces the chances of a second attack.

Vitamin E and selenium neutralise and destroy free radicals and delay the ageing process in all tissues and organs. One cause of ageing is the accumulation of free radicals over a lifetime, with associated tissue damage.

Vitamin E and selenium affect the **cardiovascular system** in many ways:

- They act as natural anticoagulants (preventing clotting of blood). This is an important fact in the prevention and treatment of diseases such as heart attacks and stroke where blood clots form in the smaller blood vessels, causing a narrowing or obstruction of the arteries.
- They improve the permeability of the capillaries (small peripheral blood vessels). This in turn improves the supply of oxygen and nutrients to all tissue, which is important in the long-term recovery after a heart attack.
- They help the blood vessels to expand so that the blood circulation improves and the blood pressure decreases in cases of high blood pressure.
- They prevent the oxidation of LDL-cholesterol – and therefore atherosclerosis.

Vitamin E and selenium also play a very important role in the treatment of diabetes. They restrict the damage of the free radicals produced as a result of the abnormal metabolism of glucose and oxygen in diabetics. They also decrease the insulin requirements of insulin-dependent diabetics and prevent damage to smaller blood vessels, a typical side effect in long-term diabetes. (Think of damage to the retina, gangrene and damage to the kidneys.)

Vitamin E and selenium are important in the prevention and treatment of breast, lung, uterine and stomach cancer. In fact, they are recommended for all types of cancer. Vitamin E improves the ability of cancer cells to differentiate again so that they start to look and act like normal cells again. This suppresses the growth of and limits the increase in cancerous cells.

Both vitamin E and selenium are recommended for people suffering from Parkinson's disease, Alzheimer's disease, epilepsy and multiple sclerosis.

Vitamin E and selenium promote the healing of wounds and reduce the formation of scar tissue. It is important to take these nutrients before and after any form of surgery, especially plastic surgery, and in the case of any skin complaints such as acne, psoriasis and eczema. They can be taken orally and applied to the skin in the form of a tissue oil.

Vitamin E and selenium are essential for a healthy immune system. They improve cell-mediated (T-cell) and humoral (B-cell) immunity. They also improve the effectiveness of phagocytes (large scavenger cells that ingest toxins and foreign organisms). They also increase the general resistance to infection.

3 L-glutathione
(About 200 mg a day on an empty stomach)

The L or D preceding an amino acid or other micronutrient refers to the molecule's ability to bend light to the right (D = dextro) or to the left (L = levo). The L form is usually the more natural form of the amino acid. If prefixed by acetyl or hydroxyl, it is a much more active and potent form of the precursor molecule. Acetyl-L-cysteine is more active than L-cysteine on its own.

The amino acids L-cysteine (500 mg a day) and N-acetyl-L-cysteine (500 mg a day on an empty stomach) are both part of the protein glutathione and both act as very potent neutralisers and scavengers of free radicals on their own. Together with glutathione and selenium, they form the extremely strong antioxidant enzyme glutathione peroxidase. L-cysteine (L-cys) and N-acetyl-L-cysteine (NAC) can be taken as separate supplements. They will be converted to glutathione in the body, along with selenium.

Vitamin C and B6 should also be taken with all amino acids. Unlike vitamins, amino acids are absorbed best when taken on an empty stomach.

Synthesis of glutathione

Glutathione peroxidase (GP) is the main antioxidant enzyme in the body. There is a good correlation between the amount of GP present and the life expectancy of a species. The higher the level of glutathione peroxidase in a specific animal species, the greater its life expectancy. The assumption that increased GP levels in humans will increase life expectancy (or delay ageing) is being thoroughly researched. The same applies to superoxide dismutase (SOD), the other important antioxidant enzyme.

If glutathione is taken as a supplement, it has to be broken down in the body into L-cys and NAC before it is converted into glutathione and ultimately GP. It is therefore advisable to take either L-cys or NAC, which is used immediately to make glutathione. Cysteine increases the GP levels in the blood and NAC with selenium gets to the root of the ageing process. It delays ageing and prevents virus infections (including AIDS) and cancer.

Glutathione peroxidase improves the detoxification of the liver and liver cells by neutralising toxins, free radicals and metabolic and hormonal waste material. It protects the body against heavy metals, air pollution, smoke, medication, preservatives, dyes and the toxins in pesticides. GP boosts the immune system and is important for maintaining the integrity of all cell membranes.

Glutathione and its two precursors (L-cys and NAC) prevent the oxidation of LDL-cholesterol and thus atherosclerosis.

Vitamin E is very important in all cardiac disorders. It also works in a complementary relationship with glutathione peroxidase. It is therefore important to take them together.

Do not underestimate the role of homocysteine (as represented in the diagram on page 70), a natural precursor to cysteine, NAC and glutathione. An accumulation of homocysteine is probably the most important factor in the onset and development of atherosclerosis – even more important than high LDL-cholesterol and low HDL-cholesterol. The reason for the accumulation of this natural intermediate step in the synthesis of glutathione is a vitamin B6 deficiency. Vitamin B12 and folic acid are also important for the conversion of homocysteine into cysteine. All adults should be checked for genetically high levels of homocysteine, as well as cholesterol. This is another essential reason for taking vitamin B6, B12 and folic acid supplements. As long as 30 years ago research proved conclusively that it is homocysteine rather than LDL-cholesterol that rapidly accelerates the process of atherosclerosis. This research, however, was suppressed by pharmaceutical companies that had donated large amounts of money to the research of the role high cholesterol played in the development of atherosclerosis.

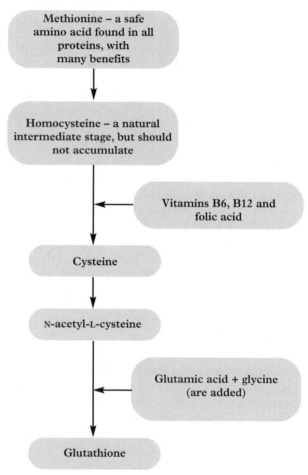

Diagram 5.2: Synthesis of glutathione

Homocysteine is also a factor in the development of cancer, osteo-porosis and Alzheimer's disease.

If L-cys, NAC or glutathione are taken as supplements, homocysteine will not be formed as the supplement provides the end products towards the final synthesis of glutathione.

The recommended dosage and combination for those suffering from cardiovascular disease or high cholesterol with atherosclerosis: Vitamin E (400 IU or 332 mg,) B6 (50 mg) and B12 (50 microgram), including folic acid (400 microgram) are the most important. They are inexpensive and easy to take. You can also include other antioxidants and NAC if you like.

4 Vitamin C
(1 500-2 000 mg; daily requirements vary – for active cancer take up to 5 000 mg a day; take vitamin C in divided doses)

This antioxidant is best known for its ability to maintain and improve the activity of the immune system. It improves the body's general resistance to all types of infection. Vitamin C concentrates in the neutrophil, the most important white blood cell which forms the first line of defence against foreign invaders. Vitamin C increases the production of lymphocytes, another type of white blood cell which is important for the production of antibodies against a number of foreign organisms and toxins. Vitamin C is therefore essential for effective protection against viruses, bacteria, parasites, fungi and carcinogens. It increases the production of interferon, an important activator in the immune system, especially for activating the immune reaction against viruses and tumour (cancer) cells (cancerous).

Micronutrients that stimulate the activity of the immune system only improve the function of mature, normal white blood cells. They do not trigger the increased formation of precursor cells. The fear of triggering cells that could cause leukaemia is unfounded. These cells are abnormal, immature precursor cells that usually have to mature in the bone marrow before they appear in the blood. In leukaemia there is an increased production of these immature cells, which circulate in the blood and suppress the maturation of other white blood cells. Antioxidants do not promote this process; they increase the number of mature cells in circulation, they improve general immunity and fight the disease process in this way.

Extensive research shows that vitamin C can be used to treat autoimmune diseases (such as rheumatoid arthritis, lupus, ulcerative colitis, Crohn's disease and Graves' disease), allergies and AIDS. There is probably a strong autoimmune component in AIDS too. Autoimmune means immune system cells attacking its own body's cells.

Vitamin C reduces the risk of atherosclerosis by ingesting free radicals and preventing the oxidation of LDL-cholesterol.

Vitamin C protects the mucosal membranes of the respiratory, digestive and urogenital systems from infection.

Vitamin C acts as a natural antihistamine, improving all types of allergic reactions by reducing the histamine levels. Histamine released by mast cells (a type of white blood cell) causes most of the symptoms in allergic reactions.

Vitamin C is probably best-known for its role in collagen production. Collagen maintains and gives structure to the subcutaneous tissue and protects the structure of the skin. Loss of collagen is an important cause in ageing of the skin. Vitamin C retards this process and improves the collagen support in the joints, vertebrae and ligaments. It is important in the prevention of sport injuries. Vitamin C is therefore vitally important for maintaining the condition of all tissues and accelerating the healing process after injury or tissue damage.

Vitamin C accelerates the detoxification of toxins in the liver. Vitamin C neutralises nitrosamines that are absorbed from the digestive tract. These commonly found carcinogens are formed when the fat from barbecued meat drips onto the coals and the resulting chemical substance is absorbed by the meat. Vitamin C protects the body against absorption of carcinogens in the digestive tract by obstructing carcinogenic absorption from the intestines and faeces.

As an antioxidant vitamin C protects the body from damage caused by free radicals. It is generally used in the prevention and treatment of all chronic diseases, especially cancer.

5 Minerals: zinc, copper and manganese
(Zinc 15 mg, copper 2 mg and manganese 10 mg a day)

These minerals are essential for a healthy immune system. They form an integral part of the body's antioxidant enzyme systems and act as co-factors. Whenever a cell has an increased need for antioxidant enzymes, when there is an increased formation of free radicals, the cell can increase the activity and quantity of these enzymes. If, however, the mineral co-factor is absent, the enzyme will be unable to function.

Marginal deficiencies of these important trace elements weaken the activity of enzymes, resulting in reduced immune function and sluggish destruction of free radicals.

6 Co-enzyme Q10
(10-20 mg twice a day)

Co-Q10 (ubiquinone) mainly acts as a support mechanism for the body's energy systems. This co-enzyme occurs in abundance in the mitochondria of every cell. The mitochondria are the power generators of the cell where all the energy for the cell's biochemical functions is produced. Energy is stored in the cell in the form of adenosine triphosphate (ATP) which is released as energy molecules when required. Co-Q10 is an essential catalyst in this process.

Co-Q10 is manufactured in all cells from the amino acids tyrosine and methionine. The required therapeutic quantities, however, are much higher than the body can produce for itself or that can be consumed from food.

Any process which accelerates the metabolism (such as stress, participation in sport or chronic diseases like diabetes) increases the energy requirements of the cells and hence the Co-Q10 requirements. Marginal deficiencies cause cells to become sluggish and function poorly. This aggravates the disease process or cell injury. Co-Q10 supplements restore the cell's energy.

Co-Q10 is a mild metabolic stimulant; it increases the body's metabolic rate. Increased metabolism requires more fuel from glucose. This is provided by the combustion of carbohydrates and fat. Co-Q10 is therefore a support mechanism for loss of body mass.

The co-enzyme is an immunostimulant and an antioxidant and it reinforces the functions of vitamin E and vice versa. One of the ways in which it boosts the immune system is by improving the activity of the macrophages (large scavenger cells in the immune system). The macrophages are then better able to destroy bacteria and tumour cells. Co-Q10 prevents atherosclerosis and is also used in the treatment of AIDS.

Co-Q10 is recommended for people with cardiovascular disease such as heart failure, arrhythmia (irregular heart beat), cardiomyopathy and after bypass procedures. It is important to take it after heart attacks, atrium fibrillation, pericarditis, cardiomyopathy, angina and high blood pressure. Co-Q10 is strongly recommended for all patients who are about to undergo cardiac surgery. Conventional prescription medication for cholesterol can reduce the Co-Q10 levels considerably. It is therefore important to take additional Co-Q10.

The production and supply of Co-Q10 in the body diminishes with age. This is why it is important to supplement as you get older.

7 Pycnogenol (proanthocyanidin)
(Up to 70 mg a day)

Proanthocyanidin supplements contain extracts of pine bark or grape seed. Pycnogenol is responsible for the aroma and taste of really fresh fruit and vegetables. It is a strong antioxidant that is particularly important in the treatment of arthritis and disorders involving poor blood circulation such as diabetes, varicose veins and cardiovascular problems.

Proanthocyanidin can penetrate the blood-brain barrier to carry out its antioxidant activity within the brain and protect brain cells from the damage of free radicals (important in Alzheimer's disease). It reinforces the capillaries and blood vessels – an important function after a stroke. It prevents atherosclerosis and is generally used for the prevention and treatment of cancer.

8 Cruciferous and carotenoid complexes

Several antioxidant combinations contain extracts of broccoli, cabbage, mustard seed, acerola cherries, cauliflower, tomato, carrot, celery, turmeric and rosemary. These are all examples of fresh fruit and vegetables in which these complexes are present in high concentrations.

Cruciferous and carotenoid complexes protect the body against cancer. They interfere in the progression phase of the cancer-triggered cell and restore the communication channels or gap junctions of cancer cells. They contain a wide range of all the most important antioxidants. (The development of cancer is illustrated in diagram 5.1 on page 64.)

Rosemary is a strong antioxidant. It acts as a carcinogen inhibitor or blocker, preventing potentially cancer-triggering substances (carcinogens) from binding to receptors on the nucleus that contains the DNA molecule. Rosemary improves the detoxification ability of the liver by improving the functioning of its carcinogen-destroying enzymes. Rosemary also acts as an anti-inflammatory agent – it prevents all types of inflammation such as arthritis, muscle injuries and myositis (inflammation of the muscles).

Curcumin, the yellow pigment in turmeric, is extremely effective against viral infections and also acts as a potent anti-inflammatory agent. Research has shown that turmeric is successful for the treatment of AIDS.

The active ingredients in carotenoids are potent phytochemicals (phyto = plant), found in the fat-soluble pigment of yellow, orange, red and green fruit and vegetables. There are more than 400 known phytochemicals, about 50 of which have provitamin A activity and are themselves potent antioxidants. Besides beta carotene, other examples are lycopene (the red pigment in tomatoes), lutein and zeaxanthin in spinach.

The cruciferous complexes are rich in antioxidants because of their high vitamin C and flavonoid content. They also contain plant chemicals such as indoles and isocyanates which neutralise carcinogens and therefore protect the body against all types of cancer, particularly cancer of the colon. Examples of cruciferous complexes are cabbage, broccoli and Brussels sprouts.

9 Bioflavonoids

Flavonoids are water-soluble phytochemicals which impart the water-soluble colour pigment to fruit, vegetables, grains, seeds, leaves and tree bark.

Grapes, grape juice and wine are rich in the flavonoids catechin and resveratrol. The anthocyanidin gives red grape skins their characteristic deep-red colour. They provide protection against cancer, atherosclerosis and other cardiovascular diseases and reduce inflammation. You always knew red wine was good for you! The French obviously know something. In all the countries where there is a high consumption of red wine the incidence of cardiovascular disease is very low, despite a high-fat diet.

Green and black tea contain catechins which provide protection against LDL-cholesterol oxidation and suppress the growth of many types of cancer. They also provide protection from the damage of free radicals caused by air pollution and smoking.

Soya beans contain isoflavones such as genistein. These bioflavonoids have low-grade oestrogen activity and protect against oestrogen-dependent cancer (breast cancer and cancer of the uterus) and prostate cancer by binding to cell receptors and preventing the body's potentially cancer-forming oestrogen from binding to them. Isoflavones are also recommended for treating symptoms of menopause.

The **onion** family, including onions, garlic, shallots and leeks contain flavonoids, vitamin C, selenium and sulphurous substances. Garlic provides protection against free radicals, prevents LDL-oxidative, provides protection against cancer and is used in the treatment and prevention of all types of infection. It improves immunity and reduces blood pressure. It acts as an expectorant (loosens phlegm) in respiratory tract infections. Garlic reduces fever and also acts as an antiseptic.

Onions contain quercetin, a bioflavonoid which acts as an expectorant in infections of the upper respiratory tract. Onions reduce blood pressure and cholesterol and prevent the formation of blood clots (in thrombosis, heart attacks and stroke). They also help to fight cancer.

10 Cat's claw *(Uncaria tomentosa)*
(100-130 mg a day)

This Peruvian herb is a potent immunostimulant and is active in the fight against viruses and suppression of cancer growth. It has a strong anti-inflammatory effect, especially after sport injuries.

Cat's claw is generally used in the treatment of cancer, arthritis, herpes infections, AIDS, allergies, peptic ulcers, diabetes, chronic fatigue, premenstrual tension, all digestive tract disorders and depression. It is the perfect panacea!

The 6-oxindol alkaloids are excellent for boosting the function of the immune system to optimal levels, while the rhyncophylline alkaloids in cat's claw help to prevent thrombosis, heart attacks and stroke by suppressing platelet aggregation (blood clotting).

11 Alpha lipoic acid (ALA)
(20-100 micrograms a day)

ALA is the subject of ongoing research because it is such a potent antioxidant and delays and retards the onset of the ageing process.

Considering the body's significant need to destroy free radicals, it produces very little ALA.

ALA is also commonly used in the treatment of diabetes and to support the liver's detoxification ability. It is effective in neutralising toxic metals, medication and other metabolites.

Spinach, liver, red meat and broccoli are excellent sources of ALA.

12 Ginkgo biloba
(120-160 mg a day in divided doses)

Ginkgo is one of the best researched herbs in the world. The leaves are shaped like the two lobes of the brain. It comes from a Chinese tree which has been in existence for 200 million years and is a living fossil.

Ginkgo has two groups of active ingredients: the ginkgo flavone glycosides and the terpene lactones. The glycosides include the bioflavonoids, the best known being quercetin, campherol and isohamnetine.

The bioflavonoids in ginkgo make it an active antioxidant in the brain and cardiovascular system. It also prevents platelet clotting and reduces the viscosity of blood; so it is less inclined to form clots. This is important in the treatment of heart attacks, thrombosis and stroke. It improves blood circulation. The antioxidant effect is very important in the brain as it is very sensitive to damage from free radicals. Brain cells have a high lipid content making it susceptible to free radical damage. This damage plays an important role in many disorders of the central nervous system associated with age, especially Alzheimer's disease and senility. It is now generally accepted that the damage caused by free radicals is more important in the deterioration of the intellectual functions in Alzheimer's disease and senility than the degeneration of the nerve tissue itself.

It is, however, the terpene lactones and the ginkgoloids and bilobaloids which hold the key to ginkgo's dramatic effects in the brain. These ingredients improve the blood circulation in the brain and in the rest of the body, providing the cells with more oxygen, glucose and other nutrients. Ginkgo also protects the nerve cells and improves memory and intellectual functions in older people who show loss of cognitive brain function. (This is the intellectual process in which knowledge is acquired, interpreted and integrated.) Ginkgoloids and bilobaloids also suppress a substance which causes damage to the nerves and reduces blood flow to the brain. This substance causes congestion in the respiratory tract and a general reduction in oxygen intake.

Ginkgo is commonly used in the treatment of cerebrovascular insufficiency, where the blood flow to the brain is reduced (such as after a stroke, in dementia, Alzheimer's disease and ischaemic incidents), and intermittent claudication (recurrent severe cramps in the calf muscles during walking or exercise). It is also used for tinnitus (ringing in the ears), vertigo (dizziness) and impotence. (Ginkgo's role in the central nervous system is discussed in detail in Chapter 11.)

13. *Rosa roxburghii*
(10 g of crystals or 10 ml of extract, three times a day)

Rosa roxburghii is a Chinese herb that has recently been released in South Africa and is the subject of intensive research here. This traditional plant is indigenous to China and contains more than 35 micronutrients.

Rosa roxburghii is particularly rich in the antioxidant enzyme superoxide dismutase (SOD) and it contains micromolecular and macromolecular SOD. This means that the body can absorb it very well. The normal SOD supplements have to be broken down into amino acids in the body before they are built up again. Micromolecular SOD combinations, however, have the ability to directly destroy superoxide free radicals.

The provisional results seem very promising. The functions of *Rosa roxburghii* include the following:

- It increases the SOD levels in the body, thereby improving the body's own ability to destroy superoxide free radicals.
- It increases glutathione levels, which improves the destruction of free radicals.
- It detoxifies the whole body.
- It reduces lipid peroxidation, one of the greatest sources of free radical production in the body, where cell membranes in particular are damaged.
- It improves the body's endurance capacity during exhaustive exercise and increases energy levels.
- It improves the body's general ability to cope with stress so that times of prolonged, intense stress are less exhausting.
- It stimulates the immune system and makes it function better.

Rosa roxburghii is rich in vitamin C and bioflavonoids. It contains vitamins A, B1, B2, D and E and the minerals calcium, magnesium, phosphorous, iron, zinc, copper, germanium, strontium and selenium. It contains all the essential amino acids that we need to take in through our diet – in fact it contains all 20 amino acids. Like red grapes with the pips and raw honey, it is an example of one of nature's most complete and perfect foods, containing all the necessary micronutrients.

Rosa roxburghii crystals and extract are recommended in particular as a natural dietary supplement for people who are suffering from any kind of stress, who exercise a lot – especially in competitive sports, and any situation where the immune system is under pressure and needs support such as AIDS, cancer, allergies and in chronic infections.

14 Vitamin B-complex
(25-100 mg plus 400 µg folic acid and 50 µg B12)

The B-complex group of vitamins act as minor antioxidants. As co-factors, however, they are essential for the effective functioning of the antioxidant enzymes.

Folic acid is essential for normal deoxyribonucleic acid (DNA) in the nucleus of every cell. Marginal deficiencies can lead to chromosome defects. Most adults have a folic acid deficiency, making supplementation essential. This is especially important in cancer where a malfunction in growth control caused by a genetically inherited DNA chromosome abnormality already exists. Vitamin B12 and folic acid reverse early changes in lung cancer.

Vitamin B6, B12 and folic acid are also very important for regulating the quantities of homocysteine. They prevent the damage to blood vessels (atherosclerosis) associated with high levels of homocysteine.

In conclusion

You should be able to make a good selection of antioxidants from the list. You are unlikely to find all the ingredients you need in one product. Look for products that contain as many of the antioxidants as possible and ensure that you do not have to take eight tablets a day to get enough of everything. Glutathione or N-acetyl-L-cysteine can be taken as a separate supplement.

Case studies

Michael Human (52) is an active, hardworking businessman with a history of increasing fatigue over the previous two years. Extensive medical examinations and tests all proved negative. His heart and lung functions were normal. Exertion (stress) electrocardiograms (ECG to test the heart muscle function while exercising) showed normal results. The liver function and blood count were within normal limits. Various tonics (some containing stimulants and caffeine) were prescribed and he was given countless vitamin B-complex injections. These treatments helped for a while, but the tonics made him feel shaky and caused insomnia.

I recommended a healthy, wholesome diet, regular walking for exercise and also some relaxation techniques every day. I prescribed a daily antioxidant combination in the suggested quantities and extra N-acetyl-L-cysteine, which he took in the morning and evening. Within two weeks Michael noticed a change in his quality of life and within three weeks the fatigue was a thing of the past. He now has boundless energy – he hasn't felt happier in years and he no longer suffers from constant colds.

Liz Combrinck (44) is a mother and wife with a demanding career. Over a period of six months she started feeling increasingly tired and run down. She kept getting colds and fever blisters and couldn't fall asleep at night. She was, however, not keen to take sleeping pills.

All the blood tests and physical examinations were normal. Liz started using a good antioxidant with additional glutathione morning and evening and a calcium and magnesium supplement with vitamin C and D in the evenings to prevent osteoporosis and to improve her sleeping pattern. She also took essential fatty acids. A wholesome, balanced diet designed to suit her personality and lifestyle, regular walks with her family and daily relaxation sessions completed the 'medication'.

Most women feel guilty if they set aside 20 minutes a day for themselves. But time to oneself to catch up and take stock is essential to restore balance in your life. You will feel better and be able to devote quality time to your family. Grant yourself that special time.

Liz's fatigue disappeared completely within two months.

Food supplements for diabetes mellitus (hyperglycaemia) and hypoglycaemia (low blood sugar)

Diabetes is a genetically inherited disease caused by a defect in the metabolism of blood sugar. There are two types, namely type 1 (juvenile onset) and type 2 (adult onset) diabetes. Only certain aspects about suitable supplements are discussed; a detailed discussion about diabetes falls beyond the scope of this book.

Type 1 diabetes manifests during childhood or puberty and sometimes in young adults (mainly before 30). Fewer than 15 per cent of diabetics have type 1 diabetes. This is a more serious form than type 2; it requires regular insulin injections and is caused mainly by an autoimmune defect. This means the body's immune system attacks and destroys its own cells – those that manufacture the hormone insulin in the pancreas. This results in an underproduction of insulin. Type 1 diabetics usually need to have insulin injections every day for the rest of their lives to control their blood sugar levels effectively. They can, however, decrease their insulin needs by taking natural supplements and making a few lifestyle changes, such as exercising. The aim for type 1 diabetics should be to try to keep their insulin requirements as low as possible and their bodies, and especially their cardiovascular system, as healthy as possible. Lifestyle changes include healthy eating habits with unrefined carbohydrates, high fibre intake, fresh vegetables and limited fruit (three a day), low intake of proteins and unsaturated fats, no alcohol (it increases the blood sugar levels), the same supplementation as for type 2 diabetics, plenty of exercise and stress management. (Consult Chapters 1 and 2.) Stress precipitates hypoglycaemic attacks and also makes it extremely difficult for diabetics to control their blood sugar levels.

Type 2 diabetes (adult) usually starts in middle age or during pregnancy. It is the more common form of diabetes (more than 85 per cent of diabetics have type 2 diabetes). With type 2 diabetes the body does produce insulin, but is unable to utilise it effectively because the insulin-dependent cells either lose their sensitivity to insulin or have too few insulin receptors. A general cause of type 2 diabetes is overweight or obesity and too little exercise. Losing just a few kilograms and moderate exercise such as walking for half an hour four times a week will improve the condition. Type 2 diabetes is inclined to occur in families. Diabetes and its complications are the third most common cause of death. Diabetes can also cause or aggravate cardiovascular disease. Cardiovascular disease is the main cause of death. Diabetes, like high blood pressure, is often a dormant disease which can cause advanced damage before it is diagnosed.

Most type 2 diabetics can control their blood sugar levels by losing weight, following a diet rich in unrefined (complex) carbohydrates and fibre, using food supplements and exercising regularly. People who have a family history of diabetes or whose blood sugar levels are marginal can prevent the disease in the same way. As with many other chronic diseases, the onset of diabetes often makes people stop and reconsider their lifestyle. Many people consider their disease to be the single most important factor which led to an improvement in their health and well-being. Stress is an important trigger in the onset of diabetes (and all other chronic diseases!). Stress management is therefore an essential part of coping with the disease.

Young girls and women with low blood sugar (hypoglycaemia) should be aware of the possibility of developing diabetes later in life. The fact that their blood sugar level drops too low is an indication of oversecretion of insulin by the pancreas. It causes cells to absorb glucose too rapidly and the blood glucose level drops, resulting in a decreased supply of glucose to the brain and other insulin dependant cells. There is thus already an abnormal glucose metabolism. Another general problem with low blood sugar is referred to as 'dumping' of blood sugar levels. If you become too hungry, your blood sugar level drops very low and you feel nauseous. So you eat a large slab of chocolate and your blood sugar level shoots sky high. The pancreas goes into top gear and secretes an oversupply of insulin. This causes your blood sugar level to drop even lower than it was before. You feel ill, listless, irritable and depressed. A few years of fluctuating glucose levels can also lead to type 2 diabetes, whereas healthy eating habits will prevent it completely from happening. Chromium is a mineral which helps keep blood sugar levels constant.

Insulin is secreted by the pancreas immediately after eating. Carbohydrates are broken down into glucose in the intestines and then transported to the liver. Some of the glucose is stored in the liver as glycogen for readily accessible glucose when energy is required. Some of the glucose is released into the bloodstream for immediate use by the organs, muscles and red blood cells. As soon as the blood sugar level increases, insulin is secreted. Insulin binds to the cell receptors and enables the glucose to enter the cell membranes of fat and muscle cells thereby providing cells with energy for all their biochemical needs. (Insulin also stimulates the synthesis of fats if there is more glucose than the cell needs.) If the pancreas produces too little insulin, the glucose level in the blood becomes too high because the glucose cannot enter the cells. Those cells which are dependent on insulin for their glucose supply starve. Other cells that do not need insulin for glucose absorption (e.g. brain cells), have an oversupply of sugar and the sugar starts to ferment, causing damage to cells and organs. Think of a person without fresh water in a lifeboat, floating on the sea from which he cannot satiate his thirst.

Brain cells do not depend on insulin for the absorbtion of glucose. The brain cells absorb the glucose directly from the blood. If the blood sugar level becomes too high, the brain is oversupplied with glucose and this can cause a coma. The high blood sugar level also damages the delicate filter mechanism in the kidneys so that more urine is excreted. The kidneys also excrete more glucose. One of the most common symptoms of diabetes is frequent urination and excessive thirst. High blood sugar levels also affect various blood components.

Useful supplements for diabetics, and people with high or low blood sugar

Take additional **fibre**, such as psyllium or guar bean fibre (two teaspoonfuls) before meals with plenty of water. Sprinkle bran over your porridge at breakfast and add it to salads and other food.

Chromium is probably the most important mineral for maintaining constant blood sugar levels. It is used for the treatment of high (hyper-) and low blood sugar levels (hypoglycaemia). Chromium forms part of the glucose tolerance factor (GTF), an important molecule in the management of carbohydrate metabolism, as it improves the functioning of insulin. GTF (and hence chromium) improves the absorption of glucose in the cells so that it can be used for generating energy. GTF binds to insulin and the cell receptors to improve the absorption of glucose, thereby reducing blood sugar levels. GTF consists of one chromium molecule, two niacin molecules (vitamin B3) and three amino acids (glycine, cysteine and glutamic acid).

Lots of people have a marginal chromium deficiency. Supplementation, especially for diabetics, is essential. Diabetics, people with high LDL-cholesterol and triglycerides and even those with marginally normal glucose tolerance levels should take about 400-600 micrograms of chromium a day in an amino acid chelation or some other organic form. Research in the United States indicates that chromium supplementation significantly reduces blood sugar levels after only two months and cholesterol levels after four months. All healthy adults should take 100-200 micrograms and children about 100 micrograms of chromium in a supplement each day.

Chromium levels tend to decline with increasing age as a result of reduced absorption from the digestive tract. This can be one cause of type 2 diabetes. One reason for the current manifestation of chromium deficiency is the low levels of chromium in the soil. Fruit and vegetables are therefore also low in chromium. The refining process of food (white sugar and flour) also reduce the chromium content, which further reduces the chromium supply in the body. A diet which places an extra burden on the digestive tract (for example old food, greasy junk food and too much sugar) also reduces the absorption of chromium.

Chromium ensures that blood glucose levels remain constant and prevents the sweet cravings that so many people have. Chromium is also important in the maintenance of a healthy cardiovascular system. It reduces the harmful LDL-cholesterol and increases the good HDL-cholesterol. (Consult Chapters 7 and 8 on cholesterol and the cardiovascular system.)

The amino acids glycine, cysteine and glutamine can also be taken as supplements: 250-500 mg of each to increase the production and function of GTF.

The abnormal glucose metabolism in diabetics results in the production of lots of free radicals due to oxidative stress. This is one of the factors that leads to many of the side effects of diabetes. Next to chromium, antioxidants are probably the most important supplements for people with high or low blood sugar levels.

Vitamin E reduces cell damage and improves the healing of diabetic wounds. Vitamin E can also reduce the insulin requirements of diabetics. Type 1 diabetics must start with 100 IU of vitamin E a day and their insulin dosage must be monitored carefully. The insulin can systematically be reduced as the vitamin E dose is increased to 400 IU a day, the recommended maintenance dosage for type 2 diabetics.

Vitamin C improves glucose tolerance and liver function. Take 500 mg of additional vitamin C twice a day.

Co-enzyme Q10 is important in the metabolism of oxygen and the production of the energy molecule ATP (adenosine triphosphate). It improves oxygen consumption at cellular level. Diabetics and people with cardiovascular disease will benefit from a Co-Q10 supplement of 30-100 mg a day.

Manganese is a relatively unknown, but essential mineral that is involved in various enzyme systems which control the metabolism of glucose and proteins, bone formation, synthesis of L-dopamine (a neurotransmitter), cholesterol and mucopolysaccharides. Marginal deficiencies are common because of soil depletion, which leads to reduced manganese in nuts and wholegrain products. Manganese is part of the antioxidant enzyme superoxide dismutase. It may improve the metabolism of glucose. Diabetics can take 4-10 mg of manganese together with 10-15 mg of iron a day as part of a multivitamin or antioxidant combination.

Flavonoids such as **quercetin** (400-800 mg), **proanthocyanidin** from the extract of grape seeds or pine bark (100 mg) and *Ginkgo biloba* (120 mg) are strongly recommended for all diabetics. They prevent damage from the free radicals caused by the abnormal glucose metabolism, they reduce the damage to peripheral blood vessels, they prevent loss of sight and protect all the organs (such as the brain) from increased blood sugar levels. Take them daily in two divided doses.

Magnesium can stimulate insulin activity. Low magnesium levels are constantly observed in diabetics. Take 400 mg of additional magnesium a day (in the evenings with calcium to ensure a better night's sleep.)

Pyridoxine (vitamin B6) can be a useful supplement, especially in improving the damage to the extremities of limbs (the feet, toes and calves) caused by poor blood circulation. Vitamin B6 also improves the oxygen supply to tissue and helps to prevent atherosclerosis (thickening of the arteries). Take 50-100 mg a day.

Vitamin B12 can also reduce the symptoms of diabetes. Take 200 micrograms a day.

Zinc supplements help to control the blood glucose levels. Take 30 mg a day.

Vanadium is another mineral involved in the metabolism of glucose which can reduce high blood glucose levels. It is used in the treatment of atherosclerosis and cardiovascular disease. Take 50 micrograms a day in a supplement.

These **medicinal herbs** can help to reduce blood glucose levels:

- Blueberry (bilberry or *Vaccium myrtillus*) is commonly used in Europe, England and America. A tea made from the leaves is a safe, mild remedy for reducing blood sugar in type 2 diabetics. Drink one cup a day for at least three months. Blueberry is also available as a tincture or extract (200 mg a day).

- Milk thistle (silymarine) is also recommended for diabetics and can be taken as a tea or two capsules three times a day.
- Fenugreek (*Trigonella foenum-graecum*, Greek hay) capsules (200 mg three times a day before meals) or tea (one teaspoon of ground seed mixed with boiling water three times a day) can reduce blood glucose levels in type 2 diabetics.
- Garlic (four capsules a day or eat plenty of fresh garlic in food) also helps to control blood sugar levels.

In conclusion

Type 2 diabetes is manageable and can be prevented by making lifestyle changes and taking supplements. It is worth giving it a try. Diabetes is a potentially life-threatening disease, but it is not the end of the world if you have it. If you are prepared to change your habits, it can be controlled. But do this under the guidance and supervision of your doctor.

Type 1 diabetics will probably always need insulin, but deep-seated emotional and psychological scars may be a contributory cause. (Your own immune system attacks its own pancreas tissue – try to find the link.) Even in type 1 diabetics correct supplementation and healthy lifestyle habits will decrease insulin requirements and improve general wellbeing.

Liver disorders

The liver is a very active organ and liver function has to be optimal for the body to remain healthy. Liver damage (such as jaundice, hepatitis, whether acute or chronic, and cirrhosis associated with alcohol abuse) is diagnosed by testing liver enzymes in the blood. These tests are only done at the request of a medical doctor. The liver has the ability to regenerate itself. Treatment of disorders is therefore aimed at allowing the liver to rest so that healthy new cells can be formed.

Hints for a healthy liver

- Follow a low-protein and low-fat diet. High-protein drinks place a great strain on the liver. Eat plenty of carbohydrates, fruit and vegetables.
- Avoid alcohol completely.
- Stop smoking.
- Try to avoid taking any medication, including over-the-counter and prescription medicine, until the liver has recovered. Most medicines are metabolised in the liver.
- Avoid all protein and amino acid supplements. Resume amino acid supplementation once the liver has recovered. It is seldom necessary to take more than one or two amino acid supplements. The amino acid l-glutathione, however, is useful as it neutralises harmful liver toxins and protects the liver. Take 250 mg a day on an empty stomach.
- Avoid environmental toxins, including petrol and exhaust fumes, smoke and pollution. Use this as a good excuse to take a break at a spa or health resort!
- Drink plenty of water and take a steam bath or a sauna to help the body get rid of toxins.
- Three herbs are of value:
  - Dandelion root tea (*Taraxacum officinale*), as often as you like, is a good diuretic. Infuse one tablespoon of the root in a cup of boiling water and drink it at least three times a day.
  - Milk thistle (*Silybum marianum* or silymarine) is a non-toxic herbal remedy which assists the regeneration of liver cells and protects the liver from toxins. Take two capsules three times a day until the liver functions are normal again.
  - The berry of the Chinese herb *Schisandra chinensis* is used to accelerate the recovery of the liver. Add two teaspoons of the dried berries to cold water, bring to the boil and simmer for 20 minutes. Strain it and drink regularly. Schisandra is often prescribed for fatigue, depression and as a general tonic.
  - Take an antioxidant combination to accelerate the detoxification process and to reduce the damage from free radicals. The liver is an active metabolic organ where large numbers of free radicals are formed. During infection or inflammation even more free radicals are formed. Bioflavonoids protect the liver against the effects of alcohol and accelerates recovery after hepatitis. (Refer to beginning of this chapter.)

6 The importance of supplements for sportsmen and -women

(In collaboration with Dr Paul van der Merwe,
specialist in sports medicine)

The whole issue surrounding the use of supplementary macronutrients and micronutrients for all athletes is still very controversial. There are almost as many opinions on this topic as there are ranges of supplements on the market. This chapter will help to separate the facts from the fiction. Follow a well-balanced daily diet using the food pyramid as a guideline.

It is useless to follow high-protein diets or take protein powders if the body has a deficiency of the co-factors or co-enzymes needed for the enzymes to break down the proteins into amino acids. The most important of these co-factors are vitamin B6, B12 and folic acid. Taking part in sport depletes these co-factors dramatically. Protein is needed for the maintenance and building of muscle tissue, but it is always better to take the amino acid building blocks of protein rather than to take proteins as such. The body can then form its own proteins as needed. If you consume proteins in the form of meat or powders, they are first broken down into amino acids, absorbed in the digestive tract, and then converted into proteins in the body. Taking amino acids from the outset means that they are rapidly absorbed and the body can use them to build muscle tissue, synovial fluid or energy as required.

High-protein diets increase the burden on the kidneys and liver, and contribute to the formation of toxic metabolic by-products in the colon and rest of the body.

Valuable amino acids for athletes

As is recommended for all amino acid supplements, they must be taken on an empty stomach together with vitamins C (250-500 mg), B6 (50-100 mg), B12 (50 micrograms) and folic acid (400 micrograms). It is unnecessary to take more than three supplementary amino acids. Sport participants must consult a medical doctor who knows about sports medicine and the use of micronutrients to ensure that the correct amino acid supplements are taken.

- L-arginine (500 mg a day on an empty stomach) is important for the production of muscle energy. It improves immunity and contributes to muscle growth and the recovery of muscles after injuries. It must not be taken by people suffering from schizophrenia or herpes infection.
- Short-chain amino acids (leucine, isoleucine and valine – about 150 mg of each on an empty stomach) are important for muscle recovery, improved muscle recovery after exercise (they serve as an alternative source of energy when glycogen in the muscles is depleted during exercise) and they also protect the muscles by improving muscle strength.
- L-carnitine (500 mg a day on an empty stomach) prevents muscle weakness and improves aerobic endurance by improving the oxygen consumption of muscles.
- L-glutamine (500 mg a day on an empty stomach) accelerates muscle recovery time and increases muscle mass. Glutamine is the most abundant amino acid in muscle tissue.
- Glycine (500 mg a day on an empty stomach) improves the synthesis of collagen (one of the main components of muscle tissue) and increases the secretion of the growth hormone that assists in muscle building.
- Gamma amino butyric acid (GABA, 500 mg a day on an empty stomach) may accelerate the release of growth hormone, thus improving muscle growth and development, according to various studies. GABA acts as an anabolic substance (for building up), without the disadvantages of anabolic steroids. It should not be used in conjunction with sedatives.
- L-ornitine (500 mg a day on an empty stomach) can stimulate the release of growth hormone, thereby promoting the synthesis of muscle tissue. It also improves energy generation in the muscles. It should not be used by people suffering from schizophrenia or herpes infections.
- Phosphatidyl serine (PS): 100 mg a day can reduce cortisol levels in athletes who train intensively and competitively. Cortisol is a catabolic hormone which accelerates the break down of muscle tissue. To succeed in sport you have to train hard. But the body responds to intensive training just as it does to any other form of stress: the adrenal glands secrete more cortisol. One of the functions of cortisol

is to maintain the blood sugar levels, which is essential for the increased energy requirements of the body during training. One way in which cortisol does this is to break down hard-earned muscle tissue proteins into amino acids which are converted into glucose in the liver. Intensive training also increases testosterone levels in men and women. Testosterone stimulates the building up of muscle tissue. During intensive training athletes should aim to achieve a balance between the muscle-building function of testosterone and the muscle-destroying function of cortisol. To achieve this some athletes resort to taking anabolic steroids which can lead to infertility, aggression, increased risk of atherosclerosis, cardiovascular disease, liver tumours and kidney disorders.

Recent clinical studies show that phosphatidyl serine, a cell membrane phospholipid obtained from soya beans and ox brain, is able to suppress the increased cortisol levels caused by intensive training. It does not have the side effects associated with anabolic steroids. Until recently plant extracts of phospholipids such as lecithin showed only trace amounts of PS. Concentrated PS used to be made from ox brain only. Many people found this unacceptable – especially in the light of the ethical objections from vegetarians and the danger of mad cow disease. New technology, however, has made a concentrated form of soya bean commercially available. This is a safe form of PS and it has no side effects. It should not be used in conjunction with anticoagulants such as warfarin on account of the danger of a possible bleeding tendency.

PS can be produced in the body, but only through a complex series of reactions which consumes a lot of energy. This is why PS is sometimes referred to as a semi-essential amino acid. Especially during any form of long-term stress (such as intensive training) the body cannot produce sufficient PS. Normal daily dietary intake of PS is seldom more than 80 mg. Therapeutic doses for athletes are 200-800 mg a day, making supplementation essential for serious athletes.

- **Trimethyl glycine (TMG):** 500 mg a day on an empty stomach. TMG is converted into dimethyl glycine (DMG) which appears to increase oxygen levels in the tissue. It is important for athletes as it increases endurance and exercise tolerance.
- **Glucosamine:** 500 mg three times a day. Glucosamine is an amino sugar found in high concentrations in cartilage, tendons and ligaments. The body can produce only a limited amount and few foods contain glucosamine in significant quantities. Athletes who place extra strain on their joints and muscles should take glucosamine sup-

plements. It is recommended for people with osteoarthritis and to prevent injuries and treat aching muscles and joints in athletes. In many parts of Europe glucosamine is replacing anti-inflammatories as first choice of treatment. It takes longer to work, but it is more effective in the long term and has none of the known side effects. Glucosamine helps to restore the gelatine shock absorbers in the joints and prevents cartilage from being broken down. It also has anti-inflammatory properties.

None of these amino acids are remotely associated with anabolic steroids. They simply improve the body's existing muscle strength and muscle-building ability.

Taking additional amino acids provides the extra building blocks for improved functioning in people whose increased rate of metabolism makes enormous demands on their body's reserves. It is unnecessary to use all of them. Try to buy amino acid combinations, even if the individual quantities may be less than those listed. Always take vitamin B6, B12, folic acid and vitamin C in conjunction with amino acids.

Antioxidants and other vitamins and minerals

Every person who participates in sport, no matter how leisurely the pace, should start the day by taking a good antioxidant combination. (Read Chapter 5 on antioxidants.) All sport activity accelerates the metabolism and make great demands on the body. Increased metabolism requires active enzyme participation and more active support from co-enzymes and co-factors, making additional minerals and vitamins essential. Antioxidants prevent the build-up of lactic acid, which causes sore and stiff muscles. Increased metabolism also requires more kilojoules to provide energy for the muscles.

Infections such as colds and flu are common among seriously competitive athletes. This is as a result of the additional strain on the immune system caused by the increased metabolism and enzyme activity. Antioxidants have a direct effect on the immune system. All athletes who take antioxidants will soon notice that they recover more quickly after competing, they seldom have infections and they have fewer muscle injuries. This is because of antioxidant support. Antioxidants also reduce tissue irritation, inflammation and loss of energy – all side effects of an accumulation of free radicals.

Calcium, magnesium and vitamin D supplements are essential for effective musculoskeletal functioning. They also decrease the risk of injuries and accelerate muscle recovery.

Chromium improves the glucose consumption of muscles and ensures a constant blood sugar level for generation of energy.

A good combination will include most of the following:
Group 1 (multivitamin/antioxidant combination)

Vitamin A
7 500 IU (2 252 micrograms or 2,25 mg of vitamin A activity or RE) a day

Beta carotene and other carotenes
25 000 IU (15 mg) a day

Vitamin E
400 IU (332 mg) a day

Selenium
200 micrograms a day

Vitamin C
1 000-2 000 mg a day in divided doses

Bioflavonoids
300 mg a day in any combination (most fruit extracts are rich in bioflavonoids). Include garlic, peppermint, orange rind, oranges and other citrus fruit, camomile, pawpaw, green and yellow peppers, broccoli, tomatoes, rose hip, quercetin, hesperidin, flavones, catechin, citrine, rutin, etc.

Vitamins B_1, B_2, B_3, B_5, B_6
About 50-75 mg of each a day

Vitamin B_{12}
50-100 micrograms

Chromium (in amino acid chelation)
300 micrograms a day

Copper
2 mg a day

Zinc
Women 20 mg a day, men 40 mg a day

Iron
Women 20 mg a day, men 10 mg a day

Manganese
10 mg a day

Molybdenum
400 micrograms a day

Potassium
1 000 mg a day

Silica
100 mg a day

} amino acid chelation or as food form combinations

Folic acid
400 micrograms

Co-enzyme Q10
30 mg a day

Group 2

Calcium (in chelation or food form)	600-900 mg before bedtime	Consult Chapter 10 on calcium and magnesium supplementation
Magnesium (in chelation or food form)	300-450 mg before bedtime	
Vitamin C	400 mg in the evenings (additional to antioxidant combination)	
Vitamin D	200-400 IU in the evenings	

Group 3

Gamma linolenic acid (in evening primrose oil)	500 mg a day	Consult Chapter 9 on essential fatty acids
Eicosapentanoic and docosahexanoic acid (in salmon oil)	300 mg a day	

Useful herbs for athletes

Herbs can be taken in the form of tablets, gelatine capsules, drops or as a herbal tea. Some are used to enhance the flavour and aroma of food.

- **Ginseng** improves endurance and stamina. It is a general tonic and helps you cope with stress. It is not a prohibited substance in sport.
- **Cayenne pepper** (chilli) is a natural stimulant that increases the metabolism and energy levels.
- **Comfrey** as an ointment or tea that accelerates the recovery after musculoskeletal injuries and also acts as an anti-inflammatory.
- **White willow bark** is the natural form of aspirin and is an effective anti-inflammatory. It can be used in tablet form for aching muscles and joints. Meadow sweet is also a good anti-inflammatory. Both herbal remedies contain natural ingredients which protect the mucous lining of the stomach and prevent the anti-inflammatory ingredients from causing irritation.
- **Bromelain** (enzyme found in pineapples) acts as an anti-inflammatory.

- **Papain** (enzyme found in pawpaws) is also an effective anti-inflammatory.
- **Echinacea** improves immunity and prevents infections. It can also be taken during infections to accelerate recovery.
- **Eucalyptus** oil or ointment is good for massaging into aching muscles.
- **Turmeric** *(Curcuma longa)* can be applied to aching muscles as an anti-inflammatory or taken orally.
- **Ginger** has numerous functions – it suppresses the inflammatory reaction, it has strong antioxidant activity and also supports the joints.
- **Kava kava** is traditionally used as a sedative and also acts as an effective muscle relaxant.

Any active sport participation leads to a considerable loss of water. Sufficient quantities of water should therefore be consumed while and after exercising. Drinking at least eight glasses of water a day will also reduce cravings for sweet and savoury things. Drink fresh or mineral water. Energy drinks can do more harm than good. Many of them upset the body's electrolyte balance, are too sweet and contain chemicals, colourants and preservatives. Diluted fruit juices can be taken while competing. Small sips of water should be taken throughout a competition or race.

It is unnecessary to take salt tablets. They upset the body's finely tuned electrolyte balance and make you thirsty. Rather use a potassium and magnesium supplement during competitions and races.

Avoid a high saturated (animal) fat diet. Use polyunsaturated and monounsaturated fats such as olive oil, grape seed oil, canola oil or linseed oil as your source of fat. Concentrate on unrefined complex carbohydrates such as wholegrain products, wheat, seeds and pulses. The muscles and liver store the glycogen (a readily available supply of glucose and energy in the liver and muscles) produced from carbohydrates and this is the most readily available source of energy for muscle contraction.

What is carbo loading?

Complex carbohydrates such as cereals, pasta and wholewheat bread increase the quantity of glycogen available for immediate energy. Four or five days before an endurance race such as a marathon, you should increase your training and reduce your carbohydrate intake to 50 per cent of your daily diet. Eat more protein such as meat and eggs, and more fat and fruit. This exhausts the supply of glycogen in your liver and muscles. Two to three days before the event, you should increase your carbohydrate intake to 75 per cent of your total daily macronutrient intake. Eat at least three large carbohydrate meals a day with a little protein and fat. This increases your supply of glycogen to maximum capacity and you will have optimal readily available glucose during the event. Fat is also a good source of energy during an event.

After the event all these macronutrients need to be replenished. Remember that athletes who suffer from chronic fatigue benefit from a high carbohydrate diet. More cereals, pasta, wholegrain bread, vegetables and fruit also improve strength and endurance.

Eat a healthy, wholesome diet, do cross-training (alternate your main sport with other sporting activities), drink plenty of water, take your supplements every day and increase your intake of supplements before, during and right after an event. Your performance will improve, you will have fewer injuries, have a speedy recovery and have less infections.

Case study

Eric Philips (25) specialises in the pentathlon and competes whenever he can. He trains hard every day. The problem is that after every event he has to spend two days in bed and he is out of action for three weeks because of muscle injuries and upper respiratory tract infections.

When this happened yet again after a competition, he consulted us in desperation. We examined him thoroughly and prescribed a personal programme suited to his needs.

With his strenuous training programme and the stress build-up before events, his metabolism needed considerable boosting. We stopped his protein supplement and prescribed four amino acid supplements (because of his strenuous training programme) namely arginine, short-chain amino acids (leucine, isoleucine and valine), phosphatidyl serine and glucosamine. We also prescribed an antioxidant combination containing ginseng, bromelain and ginger together with supplementary calcium, magnesium and essential fatty acids. We prescribed an ointment containing white willow bark, eucalyptus oil, comfrey and aloe vera for massaging into muscles before and after events and to help warm up the muscles.

To clear up the flu symptoms we prescribed Echinacea and other natural alternatives to antibiotics for 10 days.

Eric soon felt better. He was able to train harder and set a new personal best at his next pentathlon event. His endurance and performance improved. Timeout for injuries was minimal and he recovered quickly after events. The infections were a thing of the past.

7 Micronutrients that support the cardiovascular system

Cardiovascular disorders that affect the heart and circulatory systems are very common in South Africa. Every person who suffers from any form of cardiac disease or has a family history of cardiovascular problems should take supplementary micronutrients for maximum support of the heart muscle. The heart and blood vessels have to work non-stop for a lifetime. Enzyme function and metabolism in the heart are extremely active and supplementary vitamins, minerals, amino acids and essential fatty acids provide vital support.

Factors that play the greatest role in cardiovascular disease are smoking, a diet high in saturated (animal) fats, lack of exercise and high cholesterol. These are all lifestyle factors that can be controlled. Genetic factors would then seldom come into consideration.

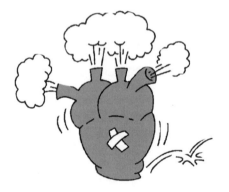

Poor lifestyle habits can place a heavy burden on the cardiovascular system. The whole system then has to work much harder to be efficient. If you don't do something about the situation and boost your cardiac function, a disease process will start.

Examples of cardiovascular abnormalities are hypertension (high blood pressure), high cholesterol with atherosclerosis, angina, varicose veins, cold (winter) hands and feet, poor circulation, heart failure, intermittent claudication (acute pain in the limbs during exercise), peripheral ulcers (open sores) on the legs on account of diabetes or varicose veins, cerebrovascular incidents and stroke. In all these instances the correct micronutrients can contribute to restored function.

All individuals who suffer from cardiovascular disease should examine their lifestyle and compile a list of priorities. This list should include correct eating habits, the use of supplements, exercise and stress management. (Consult Chapter 2 on stress management techniques.) Many patients recover completely from life-threatening cardiovascular disease after adopting a holistic approach to health.

General dietary guidelines are the same as those for general good health. The whole family will therefore benefit from them:

- Limit your intake of animal protein to twice or three times a week (this would include red meat and poultry). Stick to lean red meat such as ostrich, meat with very little fat on it (fillet) and pork. Don't eat the skin of chicken. Use herbs, lemon juice and fat-free yoghurt as flavourings and in sauces and grill meat rather than frying it.
- Try to adopt a vegetarian diet. Foods of plant origin are very low in saturated fats. Consume moderate amounts of low fat milk and yoghurt. Use olive oil, canola oil, grape seed oil and linseed oil (flax oil) in salads and cooking.
- Restrict your salt and sugar intake. Vegetable salts are a good healthy alternative to ordinary salt. A high intake of table salt (sodium chloride) plays a role only in some instances of hypertension. If you suffer from high blood pressure, eliminate salt for two weeks. If your blood pressure doesn't come down, salt is not a factor in your hypertension.
- Change to a diet similar to that of our ancestors: a high fibre diet that includes linseed oil (flax oil), oats, bran, wheat, brown rice, wholegrain products, nuts, seeds, vegetables, fruit, etc. This kind of diet provides plenty of vitamins, minerals, essential fatty acids and amino acids. It will also prevent you from getting digestive tract disorders.
- Eat onions and garlic – they protect the blood vessels and reduce cholesterol.
- Fish, especially oily fish such as trout, salmon, tuna and mackerel, are rich in omega-3 fatty acids which reduce the LDL-cholesterol and the blood pressure and protect the heart and blood vessels. Try eating fish at least twice a week.

Remember that the right kind of oils (plant and fish oils) are essential for good health. Don't eliminate all fats. You will become depressed (fatty acids are essential in the production of neurotransmitters) and your body will only start producing more of the wrong kind of cholesterol. (Consult Chapter 8 on cholesterol.)

Benefits of exercise (walking, treadmill, jogging, cycling or swimming)

- Exercise strengthens the cardiac muscle.
- Exercise improves the supply of oxygen to the heart and muscles.
- Exercise lowers the pulse rate, which reduces the load on the heart.
- Exercise reduces blood pressure.
- Exercise reduces LDL-cholesterol and triglycerides and increases HDL-cholesterol.
- Exercise reduces stress and balances the stress reaction.
- Exercise helps for depression and improves attitude to life and increases vitality.

Food supplements

1 Essential fatty acids

The recommended intake of omega-3 (in some plant oils, mainly in fish oils) and omega-6 (in vegetable oils such as olive oil and evening primrose oil) fatty acids for any cardiovascular disease is salmon oil with eicosapentanoic acid and docosahexanoic acid (1 200 mg a day) with evening primrose oil with gamma linolenic acid (2 000 mg a day). Note that the dosage is quite high for existing cardiovascular disease.

Essential fatty acids support the structure of the blood vessels and boost the activity of the heart. They are commonly recommended and prescribed for high blood pressure, high LDL-cholesterol and low HDL-cholesterol, as well as after heart attacks and stroke. They have a thinning effect on the blood and form an important part of anticoagulation therapy. (Consult Chapter 9 for more information on essential fatty acids.)

2 Antioxidants and other vitamins and minerals

Vitamin E (200-500 IU or 83-415 mg a day)

The modern diet is usually deficient in this important antioxidant vitamin. The kernel of the wheat is destroyed during the milling and refining process and most of the vitamin E is found in wheatgerm and the kernels of other whole grain products. Consuming enough vitamin E through diet alone, is virtually impossible. Vitamin E supplementation is essential. The recommended daily allowance (RDA) of 30 IU vitamin E is also totally insufficient for the body's actual needs. A disease process in the cardiovascular system dramatically increases the daily requirement of vitamin E.

Vitamin E prevents oxidation of the phospholipid chains in the cell membranes of all the cells of the body. It protects the integrity of the cell membrane. It also prevents the oxidation of the fats thereby reducing the formation of free radicals which can damage cells and tissues. This function is particularly important in the prevention of chronic inflammation of the inner lining of the arteries.

Vitamin E prevents the oxidation of LDL-cholesterol. LDL-cholesterol has to be oxidised before it can enter the arterial wall to start the process of atherosclerosis. By preventing oxidation, vitamin E ensures that LDL-cholesterol cannot penetrate the arterial walls.

The key role of vitamin E is the modification and stabilisation of fats in the blood in order to protect the arteries. This protects the heart and the whole body against the potential damage wrecked by free radicals.

Vitamin E has anticoagulation potential and prevents clots from forming within the blood vessels, as would happen in atherosclerosis, heart attacks and stroke. Abnormal blood clotting within an artery or vein also occurs in venous thrombosis (a clot in the leg) and pulmonary embolism (a blood clot moving from the legs to the lung). Vitamin E also reduces platelet aggregation, where the platelets stick to each other to form a clot. This cannot happen if vitamin E intervenes. In this respect vitamin E is more effective than aspirin.

Vitamin E is also important in preventing deterioration of varicose veins by improving the integrity of the walls of the veins.

Vitamin E improves the oxygen reserves of the cardiac and skeletal muscles by restoring the anaerobic (without oxygen) muscle function.

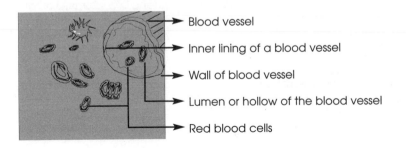

Blood vessel

Inner lining of a blood vessel

Wall of blood vessel

Lumen or hollow of the blood vessel

Red blood cells

This improves the stamina and endurance of athletes and in the case of existing cardiovascular disease or a strong family history of cardiac problems, it retards the disease process and limits the damage.

Vitamin E reduces the damage done by free radicals. Free radical formation is an inevitable part of any surgical procedure, especially cardiopulmonary by-pass operations. It also protects against the toxicity of the anaesthetic drugs.

Remember the supportive role of vitamin A for all vitamin E's functions. Take supplements of vitamin A (about 5 000 IU a day) with 20 000 IU of natural carotenes to boost the cardiovascular system.

Vitamin C (1 000-2 000 mg a day in divided doses)

Vitamin C is essential for the formation and maintenance of collagen, which forms the basis of the connective tissue in the body. Collagen supports the skin, ligaments, bones, teeth, cartilage, discs (between vertebrae), synovial lining and arterial walls. The support of the arterial walls is very important to ensure that the correct tension is maintained in the

Schematic representation of the pressure in a blood vessel (only arteries contain smooth muscle and can expand and contract).

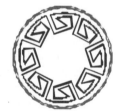

Wall of artery with layers of smooth muscle to control the tension and allow lumen to constrict and dilate.

Lumen of artery in dilated state – pressure in tube will be low and cause low blood pressure. Low blood pressure is not a disease, but the condition can be improved with supplementation for the cardiovascular system. Micronutrients improve function in a system, whether the function was overactive or underactive.

Lumen of artery in normal state – blood pressure will be normal.

Lumen of artery in constricted state – pressure in the tube will be high and the heart will have to pump the blood at a higher pressure into a narrower tube, which leads to high blood pressure.

walls of the blood vessels, a key factor in controlling blood pressure.

Vitamin C improves the excretion of LDL-cholesterol in the liver and colon, thereby reducing blood cholesterol. Vitamin C is commonly used for the prevention and treatment of atherosclerosis and helps to reduce the risk and damage of cardiovascular disease. Vitamin C increases the HDL-cholesterol and reduces the LDL-cholesterol and triglycerides.

Vitamin C is also an important antioxidant vitamin that prevents the oxidative of water-soluble molecules. It reduces the formation of free radicals that damage cells that then may lead to the onset of disease processes. Existing disease processes generate and cause an accumulation of free radicals that aggravate the disease process. Vitamin C will prevent or reduce this accumulation of free radicals. It will also protect the fat-soluble vitamins (A, D, E and K) and the B-complex vitamins from oxidation. They will therefore be able to work more effectively and for longer. Vitamin C acts as a detoxifying substance and reduces the side effects of cortisone, aspirin and insulin.

Vitamin C stimulates the immune system by increasing the production of neutrophils and lymphocytes. Both are important adult white blood cells that protect the body against foreign invaders. For this function and its antioxidant activity, vitamin C can be effectively used in

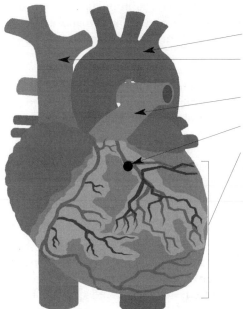

Aorta

Vena cava

Pulmonary artery

Blood clot in left coronary artery

The area beyond the obstruction (distal to the obstruction) will form large numbers of free radicals, get no nutrients and oxygen and die if no new blood vessels develop (reperfusion). Vitamins C and E help with this. They restrict the damage of free radicals and the rest of the heart can again get nutrients, work again and compensate excellently for the area that was damaged by the heart attack.

treating all chronic diseases including cardiovascular disease and cancer.

Vitamin C, together with vitamin E (and supported by vitamin A), contributes to the prevention of blood clots forming in the heart and blood vessels and helps to dissolve existing clots. Vitamins E and C prevent additional damage to the cardiac muscles and scarring after a heart attack and improve the development of collateral blood vessels (the formation of new blood vessels to transport the blood past the damaged tissue to the tissue beyond the obstruction). Vitamin C also improves the blood circulation by dilating the capillaries (the fine network of blood vessels that are in direct contact with the tissues).

B-complex vitamins

Vitamin B1 (thiamine, 50-100 mg a day) prevents the accumulation of fatty deposits in the arterial walls and so prevents the onset of and deterioration associated with atherosclerosis. Vitamin B1 also has a moderate diuretic effect and alleviates the tendency to fluid retention that is associated with many cardiovascular diseases. It boosts the cardiac function and forms part of many treatment regimes for cardiovascular disease.

Vitamin B2 (riboflavin, 50-100 mg a day) is important for cellular respiration (exchange of oxygen and carbon dioxide) and helps to improve the cell's utilisation of oxygen. This is an important aspect in maintaining cardiac function.

Vitamin B3 (niacin or nicotinic acid, 50-100 mg a day) reduces LDL-cholesterol and triglycerides in the blood and helps to dilate the blood vessels in the heart. The other molecule that is included as part of the B3 group, namely niacinamide, does not decrease (or lower) cholesterol levels. Niacinamide is the B3 vitamin mostly used in supplements. It has no side effects. High dosages of niacin (nicotinic acid) can cause toxicity of the liver (much higher doses than are recommended here) and should be prescribed under a doctor's supervision, with regular testing of liver enzymes.

Vitamin B5 (pantothenic acid, 50-100 mg a day) is important for the metabolism of cholesterol and ensures the correct balance between LDL and HDL-cholesterol. It improves metabolism and ensures an adequate supply of energy and oxygen to all the cells of the body, including the cardiovascular system.

Vitamin B6 (pyridoxine, 50-100 mg a day) is important for the production of red blood cells (the red blood cells transport oxygen to all the cells of the body), fluid and electrolyte balance and the electrical impulse conduction of the heart, nerves and muscles. It also has a diuretic effect and assists the body in getting rid of excess fluids and in controlling blood pressure.

Vitamins B6, B12 and folic acid are essential for neutralising homocysteine, a precursor of methionine. Methionine is an amino acid that is found in great quantities in red meat, milk and dairy products.

If homocysteine accumulates, as would happen with a vitamin B6 deficiency, it is very harmful to the blood vessels. It damages the endothelial lining of the blood vessels and contributes to the process of atherosclerosis.

A genetic tendency to homocysteine accumulation appears to be a more important factor in the development of cardiovascular disease than cholesterol. When a patient is checked for cardiovascular disease, it is important to also check the homocysteine levels in the blood. (Consult Chapter 5 on antioxidants.)

Vitamin B12 (50 micrograms a day) and **folic acid** (400 micrograms a day) are important for the formation of red blood cells and for neutralising homocysteine and thus contribute to the reduction of atherosclerosis. Folic acid alleviates ischaemia (an inadequate supply of oxygen to the heart) by increasing the blood flow in patients who suffer from circulatory disorders.

Inositol (50 mg a day) is also a B-complex vitamin and it plays an important role in the maintenance of the cell membrane's integrity and structure. It is used in the treatment and prevention of atherosclerosis and to reduce cholesterol.

Co-enzyme Q10
(50 mg twice a day)

Co-Q10 is a vitamin that functions as a co-enzyme. It provides protection against atherosclerosis by preventing the formation of oxidised LDL-cholesterol.

Co-Q10 is an essential part of the mitochondria (power generators of cells). A diseased heart has less Co-Q10 than a healthy heart. Supplements of Co-Q10 are valuable in the treatment of all cardiovascular diseases. Some studies indicate that with Co-Q10 supplementation the condition of heart patients can improve clinically by up to 80 per cent. It also protects the heart before and after by-pass surgery.

Magnesium in an amino acid chelation
(300-450 mg a day)

Magnesium may very well be the most important mineral for the protection of the cardiovascular system. Magnesium is essential for cardiac function and the general health of heart tissue. It relaxes the smooth muscle in the walls of the arteries and thus contributes directly to the reduction of blood pressure and the relief of angina. Magnesium also improves collateral blood flow after a heart attack. It normalises the heartbeat and is valuable in the treatment and prevention of arrhythmia (abnormal heartbeat when the electrical conduction in the heart is disturbed).

Magnesium also ensures that calcium remains in circulation so that it does not accumulate in the tissues. This is an important factor in the onset of atherosclerosis and kidney stones where abnormal forms of calcium can be deposited and then calcify.

Magnesium and calcium together are responsible for the stability of the cardiac muscles. Both are good sedatives and help the nervous system and muscles to relax properly.

Calcium in an amino acid chelation
(600-900 mg a day)

Calcium and magnesium work together. Calcium is also involved in lowering cholesterol and reducing platelet aggregation (blood clotting).

Chromium in an amino acid chelation
(200-300 micrograms a day)

Chromium plays a role in reducing levels of LDL-cholesterol. It is also important in controlling blood sugar as part of the glucose tolerance factor (GTF). The heart depends on constant blood sugar levels for its energy requirements. (Consult Chapter 5 for more information on diabetes.)

Potassium in an amino acid chelation
(150-200 mg a day)

Potassium is a very important mineral for maintaining the electrolyte and fluid balance in the body. Together with sodium it keeps the acid-base balance (pH) constant for internal homeostasis (perfect balance and harmony).

Potassium is essential for cardiovascular function and as a supplement for the treatment of hypertension. Diuretic therapy often leads to excessive loss of potassium in the urine, which can lead to a potassium deficiency.

Selenium
(100-200 micrograms a day)

Vitamin E and selenium always work together. They form part of the antioxidant system that protects cell membranes and the intracellular structures against lipid peroxidation (formation of lipid free radicals). They reduce the hardening of tissue, which is especially important in the prevention of atherosclerosis (thickening of arterial walls). It is used with great success in patients with cardiomyopathy (diseases of the cardiac muscle) and heart failure.

Zinc, copper and iron
(Zinc 15-30 mg a day, copper 2 mg a day, iron 15 mg a day)

These three minerals all form part of the structure and function of various antioxidant enzymes and are therefore important in limiting the damage from free radicals. Zinc boosts the immune function and accelerates the recovery of damaged tissue. Iron is important for the formation of haemoglobin in red blood cells. Haemoglobin transports the oxygen molecules to all the cells. Iron is also important in maintaining the inner lining of the blood vessels.

3 Amino acids that support cardiovascular function

L-carnitine
(500-1 000 mg a day on an empty stomach)

Carnitine is very important for the normal functioning of the cardiac muscle and blood vessels. It also reduces LDL-cholesterol and increases HDL-cholesterol. It is often used in the treatment of atherosclerosis, angina, cardiomyopathy, arrhythmia and as an aid to weight loss.

L-taurine
(500 mg a day on an empty stomach)

Taurine plays an important role in the regulation of the transport of minerals in and out of the cells of the cardiovascular system. It is thus essential for the electrolyte balance of potassium, sodium, magnesium and calcium. It promotes the retention of potassium and magnesium in the cardiac muscle and thus helps to normalise heart rate and contraction. Taurine also suppresses angiotensin, a protein in the blood that causes high blood pressure. It is therefore recommended in the treatment of high blood pressure, cardiomyopathy and arrhythmia.

Taurine increases the production of taurocholate, a substance that increases the excretion of cholesterol in the bile. This has the effect of lowering LDL-cholesterol.

Taurine also has a calming effect on the nervous system, an important factor in stress management.

n-acetyl-l-cysteine (NAC)
(500 mg a day on an empty stomach)

NAC is a very effective antioxidant. Together with glutathione and on its own it is an excellent scavenger of free radicals. It also forms part of the potent antioxidant enzyme glutathione peroxidase.

NAC is an excellent protector of the cardiovascular system. It prevents oxidation of LDL-cholesterol and hence atherosclerosis. NAC also lowers lipoprotein A, which can be a greater triggering factor in the onset of atherosclerosis than LDL-cholesterol and trigliserides.

4 Medicinal herbs that support the cardiovascular system

- **Garlic** (four capsules a day or use fresh in food preparation) reduces platelet aggregation and therefore has the effect of thinning the blood so that clots in the blood vessels dissolve and do not form again. Garlic reduces blood pressure and cholesterol levels. Onions and cayenne pepper have a similar, milder effect.
- ***Ginkgo biloba*** (120 mg a day) reinforces the arterial walls and improves blood circulation. As an antioxidant, ginkgo also prevents oxidation of LDL-cholesterol and protects the blood vessels from damage by free radicals. It is excellent for any obstruction in the peripheral blood flow such as in Raynaud's disease, intermittent

claudication, impotence, leg ulcers due to severe varicose veins, stroke, etc. (see page 71 and 137).

- **Hawthorn berry** (*Crateagus oxyacantha*, 750 mg a day) is commonly used in Europe for the treatment of cardiovascular disease. It prevents angina and lowers blood pressure and cholesterol levels. It is an effective diuretic for the treatment of fluid retention (edema). It is used in Ayurveda (the ancient medicine of India) to treat angina and intermittent claudication to improve the blood flow to the heart, for heart failure and for high and low blood pressure. It also lowers cholesterol levels.
- **Plant oestrogens** such as found in soya beans and soya products reduce blood cholesterol.
- **Ginseng** lowers cholesterol and blood pressure and provides more energy.

Case study

Jack Simmons (47) had a heart attack two years ago. There were no warning signs. He had a stressful job; he was a perfectionist and a complete workaholic. He often worked a 12 hour day. In the evenings he would greet his wife and children, eat his supper, watch the news and then disappear into the study to work until two in the morning. He did no exercise and ate very little fresh fruit and vegetables. His father and brother both suffered from high blood pressure. Jack had a routine medical examination once a year – a company requirement for top management. Each time his ECG, blood pressure and cholesterol were normal, but he was advised to try to lose 15 kg. He did not have time to bother with that.

Then came the heart attack – an enormous blow! In the hospital he decided he would have to change his lifestyle. He realised how important his wife and children were to him and how shamefully he had neglected them. He resigned from his job and started his own business as a consultant (something he had always dreamed about). He now has a new lifestyle – an eight-hour working day, time set aside each day for meditation, walking and aerobic exercise, and he makes time to relax with his family.

After consultation he began to follow a healthy, balanced diet containing at least three fresh fruit and five vegetable portions a day, very little red meat, alcohol in moderation and much more chicken and fresh fish. In addition he started taking essential fatty acids, a calcium and magnesium supplement and a good supplement to support the cardio-vascular system. Within six months he was healthy and he no longer needed to take the blood pressure and cholesterol medication that had been prescribed after the heart attack. He now has boundless energy, his body mass is within normal limits and the children have a brand-new dad. He has experienced no more cardiovascular problems.

Warning: Never stop taking prescribed medication without your doctor's approval and supervision.

8 Cholesterol as an example of a lifestyle disease

South Africans are acutely aware of the cholesterol issue which is a genetic problem in many South African families. The whole cholesterol story has been distorted and people dread hearing the 'C' word.

Not all cholesterol is bad. It is essential for life. Cholesterol is the central molecule for the stress and sex hormones. The stress hormone is cortisol and the sex hormones include oestrogen and progesterone in women and testosterone in men. Cholesterol also forms part of all cell membranes. If we had no cell membranes, we would be shapeless puddles of jelly! Cholesterol is essential for the structure, integrity and maintenance of all the cell membranes which surround every cell in the body. Normal cholesterol medication has many side effects because it also affects the cholesterol that is essential to life.

Most of the cholesterol is produced in the body. The diet only provides about 20-30 per cent of the body's total cholesterol content. If the dietary intake of cholesterol is dramatically reduced, the body will produce more cholesterol. It is no good cutting out all cholesterol in the diet. This only leads to depression and we struggle to eat the tasteless, flavourless food. Eating is supposed to be a pleasurable activity, not a punishment. While we should try to eliminate saturated animals fats from our diet, a totally fat-free diet is counterproductive. Unsaturated plant oils are needed to keep the cholesterol in balance.

The fats in our food are broken down to fatty acids and gliserol, absorbed from the small intestine and then transported to the liver (see illustration on page 112). Only 20-30 per cent of the cholesterol comes from the food we eat. The rest is produced in the liver. The cholesterol is used to transport fats to all parts of the body to provide energy for other bodily functions. It is used for the maintenance, operation and integrity of cell membranes and, even more important, the manufacture of the steroid hormones that are essential to life (such as the sex hormones and cortisol).

The cholesterol that is digested with the fats or produced in the liver is made up in the liver into little parcels called lipoproteins. The lipoproteins consist of lipids (fats and cholesterol) and proteins. There are three kinds of lipoproteins (illustrated on page 112; explained on page 113).

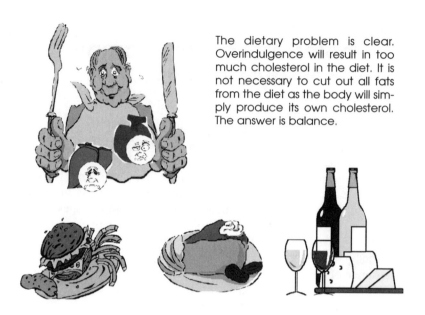

The dietary problem is clear. Overindulgence will result in too much cholesterol in the diet. It is not necessary to cut out all fats from the diet as the body will simply produce its own cholesterol. The answer is balance.

The three kinds of lipoproteins (explained on page 113):

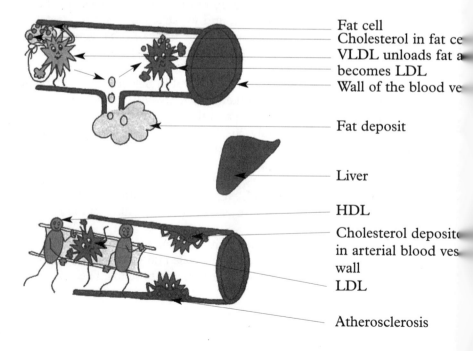

Fat cell
Cholesterol in fat ce
VLDL unloads fat a
becomes LDL
Wall of the blood ve

Fat deposit

Liver

HDL

Cholesterol deposit
in arterial blood ves
wall
LDL

Atherosclerosis

- Very low density lipoprotein (VLDL), which transports large quantities of cholesterol from the liver to other parts of the body. Too much VLDL is a problem in families with a history of high cholesterol.
- Low density lipoprotein (LDL). The VLDL offloads the fat in fat storage areas and becomes LDL. If there is too much LDL, as happens in families with high cholesterol, pieces of LDL attach themselves to the arteries, eat into the walls of the arteries and start the process of atherosclerosis (thickening of the arteries).
- High density lipoprotein (HDL). The HDL detaches the LDL from the arterial walls and clears the LDL out of the bloodstream. The HDL takes the LDL back to the liver for recirculation or excretion through the alimentary canal.

Too much VLDL and LDL (as found in a diet very high in saturated fats or families with very high cholesterol levels) result in an imbalance between LDL and HDL. The HDL is then not able to remove all the LDL that is attached to the walls of the arteries. In due course this leads to atherosclerosis or thickening of the arteries. If the first artery to become totally clogged is in the heart, it will cause a heart attack. If the first artery to become totally clogged is in the brain, it will cause a stroke.

Remember that the artery that becomes clogged is only the tip of the iceberg. Many other blood vessels have already thickened and are becoming clogged to a greater or lesser extent.

It is not only LDL that plays a role in atherosclerosis. High blood pressure, high homocysteine levels, poor stress management, lack of exercise, smoking and too much alcohol are also important factors. They can all, however, be addressed by making lifestyle adjustments.

Which factors lead to an increased risk of having too much 'bad' LDL-cholesterol and hence a good chance of developing atherosclerosis?

- Genetic susceptibility – family history
- A woman over 55 years old or a man over 45 years old

} The only two factors we cannot control

- High stress levels with poor stress management
- A diet high in saturated fats
- Smoking
- High alcohol consumption (more than two or three drinks a day)
- High blood pressure
- Lack of exercise

} We can control all these factors.

If we make lifestyle adjustments, the first two factors won't even come into consideration.

Cholesterol is used as an example of a disease where adaptations in lifestyle can make a great difference to general health and wellbeing.

Any modern chronic disease can be treated in much the same way.

Natural lifestyle management of high LDL-cholesterol

- Manage your stress levels (consult Chapters 1 and 2).
- Check your homocysteine, blood pressure and cholesterol levels regularly. This will also give an indication of how successfully you are managing your stress. (Refer to page 40 for list of medical screening tests.)
- Limit your intake of animal fats (saturated and trans fatty acids). Choose the correct monounsaturated and polyunsaturated fats in moderate amounts. Make olive oil your main source of fat intake.
- Ensure that your diet is high in fibre, unrefined wholegrain carbohydrates (such as brown rice, cereals, pulses, seeds, oats, potatoes and wholewheat bread), fresh fruit and vegetables.
- Take food supplements (antioxidants and essential fatty acids) – consult the relevant chapters. Antioxidants prevent the oxidation of harmful LDL-cholesterol and in this way stop the cholesterol from eating into the walls of the arteries and causing the onset of atherosclerosis. Essential fatty acids such as evening primrose oil, olive oil, linseed oil and salmon oil reduce the LDL-cholesterol and increase the HDL-cholesterol (the good one). This value can be measured by doing regular cholesterol tests as proof that essential fatty acids do reduce LDL-cholesterol levels and increase HDL-cholesterol.
- Eat plenty of garlic, either in your food or in capsule form with parsley. It lowers the LDL-cholesterol and total cholesterol and improves the ratio between the HDL and LDL-cholesterol.
- Give up smoking.
- Consume less alcohol – no more than two or three drinks a day.
- Exercise regularly. It increases the 'good' HDL-cholesterol, assists in weight loss and weight management, reduces stress levels, and

improves symptoms of depression and anxiety or tension. Do aerobic exercise (where the muscles use oxygen) for half an hour four times a week or 20 minutes every day. Good examples are power walking, swimming, cycling, or jogging. If you are walking, your pace should allow you to hold a normal conversation without becoming breathless. Your maximum pulse rate should be 60 per cent of your maximum heart rate for 20 minutes of your exercise period. Do some stretching before exercises and start gradually to prevent sprains and strain.

Age	Maximum pulse rate (beats per minute)	Target pulse rate (beats per minute) while walking	Target pulse rate (beats per 10 seconds) while walking
20-30	200	120-180	20-30
30-39	190	114-168	19-28
40-49	180	108-162	18-27
50-59	170	102-150	17-25
60-69	160	96-144	16-24
70+	150	90-132	15-22

Remember: Nature provides balance.
Walk in the fresh air.

Case study

Mr J. Kruger (49) had a total cholesterol count of 7,2 mmol per litre (normal is 4,5-4,9 mmol per litre). He had already been following a strict low-fat and low-cholesterol diet for six months. He exercised, but not regularly enough. Mr Kruger was unwilling to take the conventional cholesterol medication that his family doctor prescribed – especially after reading the package insert in a friend's medication and finding out about the side effects. He didn't want to risk being one of the 70 per cent of people who develop some of the many side effects of the medication.

After a general examination, exercise electrocardiogram (ECG) and advice on lifestyle adjustments and diet (we actually added more polyunsaturated fats such as olive oil to the diet he had been following so strictly without much success), we also added the following supplements:

- Omega-6 fatty acids (500 mg of evening primrose oil morning and evening, or 1 000 mg a day).
- Omega-3 fatty acids (250 mg of salmon oil morning and evening, or 500 mg a day).
- An antioxidant combination with vitamins A, E, C and B-complex; the minerals zinc, selenium and copper; plant extracts of grape seed, grape skins, turmeric, garlic, cat's claw and the co-enzyme Q10. The amounts of each are not that important, except for vitamin E, which must be at least 200 IU a day. (Use the other recommended dosages as discussed in Chapter 5 on antioxidants).

Within six weeks Mr Kruger's total cholesterol count was down to 5,5 mmol per litre and after 12 weeks it was normal (4,8 mmol per litre). He felt wonderful. His blood pressure also came down from 140/90 (higher than the upper limit of normal) to 130/80 (normal). His fatigue was a thing of the past.

He was much happier with his diet, which was not as strict and allowed him a greater variety of foods. He could manage a low intake of saturated fats and moderate intake of monounsaturated and polyunsaturated fats. (Consult Chapter 9 on essential fatty acids.)

Mr Kruger was a very satisfied and grateful patient.

9 Essential fatty acids

Poly- and mono-unsaturated fatty acids form part of the fats (lipids) that serve as a source of energy in the body; fat is the form in which the body stores its energy. Lipids also form part of the phospholipid structure of all cell membranes.

Two essential fatty acids that are not made in the body and have to be taken in with food are alpha linolenic acid (ALA), an omega-3 fatty acid, and linoleic acid, an omega-6 fatty acid.

Specific enzymes in the body convert the ALA into eicosapentanoic acid (EPA) and docosahexanoic acid (DHA). This conversion is slow and restricted in the human body. Too many omega-6 fatty acids in the diet can also slow down this conversion.

Linoleic acid can be stored in the body, oxidised to provide energy or converted into other substances such as gamma linolenic acid (GLA) and arachidonic acid which have important physiological functions in the body.

In the human body the omega-3 and omega-6 fatty acids follow two different metabolic pathways which are controlled by the same enzymes. The important tempo regulating enzyme in this process is delta-6 desaturase.

Examples of plants that are rich in ALA are the green leafy vegetables, linseeds (flax), canola and soya beans. Most omega-3 fatty acids, however, are produced by the phytoplankton (microscopically small plants) in water. They are passed into the food chain by shrimps, etc. to the higher order animals such as shellfish, seals, whales, trout, salmon, tuna, mackerel, sardines and galjoen (damba). Humans take in omega-3 when they consume any of these coldwater fatty fish (seawater and freshwater fish).

Diagram 9.1: Metabolic pathways of the omega-6 and omega-3 fatty acids

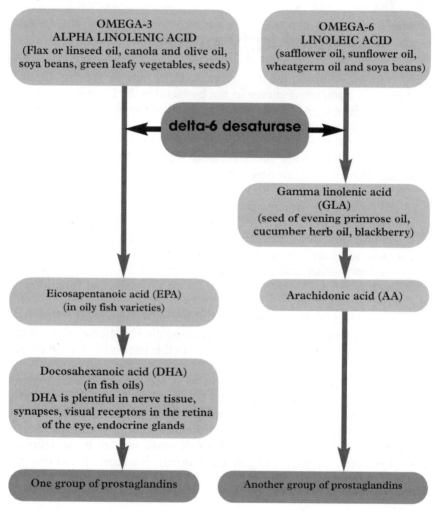

Omega-3 and omega-6 fatty acids

Omega-6 is found in abundance in plants. Olive oil and wheatgerm, cotton seed, safflower and soya beans are rich in linoleic acid. The main sources of GLA are evening primrose oil, starflower oil, borage and blackberry seeds.

Omega-3 food chain
❶ The plankton produce the omega-3 fatty acids.
❷ The shrimp eat the plankton.
❸ Other fish eat the plankton and the shrimp.
❹ The rainbow trout eat the other fish.
❺ The person catches the fish.
❻ The person eats the fish and consumes omega-3 fatty acids.

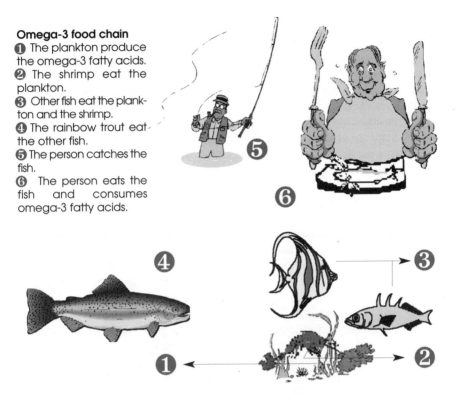

The diet of earlier generations was rich in omega-3 and omega-6 fatty acids. The typical Western diet contains mainly omega-6 fatty acids in the form of linoleic acid, with very small quantities of omega-3 fatty acids. This imbalance places a physiological burden on the human body which the specie has not yet had the time to adapt to and prepare for through genetic modification. It is therefore important to supplement the human diet with GLA, a further step in the omega-6 conversion, as well as EPA and DHA (omega-3 fatty acids) in the form of fish oil such as salmon oil. To take in a sufficient quantity in the diet alone, you would need to eat about 1 kg of oily fish a week.

Children and teenagers, people who are stressed (all of us!), pregnant women and those affected by depression, allergies, attention deficit disorder (hyperactivity), poor concentration or poor memory usually have marginal deficiencies of these essential fatty acids.

This lack is also common after injury, during infection and in people who have digestive tract problems. The needs of the foetus and the new-born baby for essential fatty acids are particularly great.

Many people have an inherited lack of delta-6 desaturase – or a weakened function of this enzyme. They are thus not able to further metabolise the ALA and linoleic acid in sufficient quantities. This is particularly noticeable in children who suffer from hyperactivity, allergies and eczema and those who suffer from diabetes, depression, poor concentration and poor memory. Prolonged and chronic stress also places great demands on the enzyme and as a person gets older the enzyme becomes less active. By taking supplements of GLA, EPA and DHA, you bypass the enzyme problem and provide the next steps in the metabolic pathways of the omega-3 and omega-6 fatty acids.

The quantities of omega-3 and omega-6 that you take are also important. In humans the two pathways are separate, but they compete for the same enzymes. If you take in too much omega-6 on its own, too little EPA and DHA will be formed. This has many health implications. The optimal intake has not yet been determined, but the National Academy of Food Sciences in the United States recommends a ratio of between 10:1 and 3:1 of omega-6 to omega-3.

The recommended supplementary intake is as follows (you also obtain essential fatty acids through the food you eat):

Pure gamma linolenic acid (GLA) (250 mg a day) or evening primrose oil (1 000 mg a day will also contain enough GLA) together with the omega-3 fatty acids of about 300-500 mg eicosapentaenoic acid (EPA) and docosahexanoic acid (DHA), such as found in salmon oil. This is only a very general indication for a daily maintenance intake. Requirements increase with any form of chronic disease, disorder of the nervous system or allergy. If your intake is greater than this, it will do no harm as long as the ratio of omega-6 to omega-3 is correct. If you replace saturated fats in the diet with monounsaturated and polyunsaturated fats, you will automatically get more omega-3 and omega-6 fatty acids. It is important to simultaneously take in more vitamin E as well (100 IU). By taking antioxidants, you will be doing this in any case. Vitamin B6, magnesium and zinc are also important co-factors for the enzymes responsible for fatty acid metabolism.

Apart from being an essential part of the phospholipid structure of cell membranes, the omega-6 fatty acids are also precursors of prostaglandins. GLA is quickly converted to dihomogamma linolenic acid (DGLA) and then prostaglandins. Prostaglandins suppress platelet aggregation thereby preventing blood clotting, an important function in the prevention and treatment of heart attacks and stroke. GLA and DGLA also suppress the inflammatory process, for example after injury, in contact dermatitis, arthritis and other joint infections. GLA and DGLA are also used to reduce blood pressure in hypertension, to decrease LDL-cholesterol and increase HDL-cholesterol. The omega-3 fatty acids form part of the phospholipid structure of cell membranes. This function of the omega-3 and omega-6 fatty acids is an important part of transfer of fluid through cell membranes, electrolyte balance, hormone function and the immune function. Some of the omega-3 fatty acids, especially EPA, are also precursors of prostaglandins. EPA and DHA play a role in the prevention and treatment of cardiovascular disease such as hypertension, high LDL-cholesterol, stroke and heart attacks.

Functions of prostaglandins, omega-3 and omega-6 fatty acids

Prostaglandins are hormone-like compounds with many functions found in all cells of the body. Biologically they are very active and form part of most biochemical activities that occur in all the organs of the body. Prostaglandins are also involved in the immune system where one of their functions is to suppress and prevent allergic reactions. This important group is also closely associated in the process of nerve transmission in the memory and concentration centres of the brain.

Apart from some of the omega-3 and omega-6 fatty acids being converted to prostaglandins, they have functions of their own. Deficiencies of essential fatty acids (EFA) are common and usually quite subtle and imperceptible.

The functions of essential fatty acids include the following:

- Essential fatty acids maintain the fluidity of all cell membranes – to ensure that fluids, nutrients and oxygen can move into, and waste products out of cells.
- Essential fatty acids help the red blood cells in transporting oxygen to cells.
- Essential fatty acids prevent blood platelets from sticking together. This prevents the blood in the blood vessels from clotting, as happens in atherosclerosis, after heart attacks and stroke, thrombosis and pulmonary embolism. As the name suggests, essential fatty acids

are crucial in the prevention and treatment of all diseases of the heart and blood vessels.

● Essential fatty acids ensure optimal and efficient kidney function.

● All the essential fatty acids are a good reserve energy source for the whole body and the main source of energy for cardiac function.

● Prostaglandins and essential fatty acids form an important part of the nervous system's neurotransmitters. They improve the release of neurotransmitters, particularly in the memory and concentration centres of the brain. Prostaglandins act as neurotransmitters themselves. Many people have insufficient quantities and/or a poor quality of the enzyme delta-6 desaturase, with the result that too little omega-6 and especially omega-3 fatty acids are produced. One of the effects is attention deficit disorder, poor concentration and all forms of hyperactivity. Poor message transfer is also a problem in depression, tension, Alzheimer's disease and other disorders of the nervous

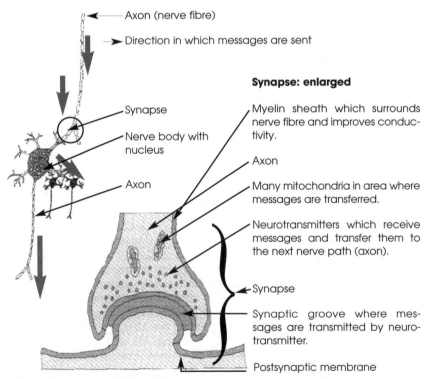

Axon (nerve fibre)

Direction in which messages are sent

Synapse

Nerve body with nucleus

Axon

Synapse: enlarged

Myelin sheath which surrounds nerve fibre and improves conductivity.

Axon

Many mitochondria in area where messages are transferred.

Neurotransmitters which receive messages and transfer them to the next nerve path (axon).

Synapse

Synaptic groove where messages are transmitted by neurotransmitter.

Postsynaptic membrane

Schematic representation of the movement of messages along an axon through a synapse to the next nerve fibre.

system such as multiple sclerosis, tinnitus (ringing in the ears) and in migraines. Essential fatty acids can also play a role in the treatment of schizophrenia. The omega-3 fatty acid docosahexanoic acid (DHA) is very important for the normal functioning of the nervous system. It is plentiful in the synapses, the points where the dendrites and neurons meet and where messages are passed from one nerve to the other by means of the neurotransmitters. DHA is essential for normal vision, as it is abundant in the retina of the eye. It is also important for normal brain and cognitive development in children and the developing embryo and foetus. (Consult Chapter 12 on the nervous system for information on the other micronutrients that play a role in the normal functioning of nerve transfer and the maintenance of the nervous system.)

That is why the condition of children and adults who suffer from allergies, poor concentration, poor memory and hyperactivity improves after taking supplements of omega-3 and omega-6 fatty acids. The problem is often a deficiency of the enzyme delta-6 desaturase. The production of prostaglandins in such cases is insufficient for the body's needs and a marginal deficiency of prostaglandins will arise in due course. By bypassing the enzyme deficiency and supplementing with the essential fatty acids, you can provide the next steps in the manufacturing process of prostaglandins. (Look at the diagram on the metabolic pathways of the omega-3 and omega-6 fatty acids on page 118.)

- Essential fatty acids and prostaglandins reduce high blood pressure by improving the smooth muscle tone in the arteries.
- Essential fatty acids decrease bad LDL-cholesterol and increase good HDL-cholesterol levels.
- Gamma linolenic acid and the omega-3 fatty acids suppress the growth of cancer cells. Tumour cells lack delta-6 desaturase, which means a lack of GLA and omega-3 fatty acids. Essential fatty acids are thus important in the prevention and treatment of all forms of cancer.
- Essential fatty acids boost the immune system and play an important role in the prevention and treatment of acute and chronic infections as well as autoimmune diseases such as rheumatoid arthritis, lupus, multiple sclerosis, ulcerative colitis and Crohn's disease. They are also important in all instances of allergy because they reduce the immune system's hypersensitivity to allergens (substances that induce an allergic reaction in sensitive people). Research has shown that people who suffer from atopic (allergic) eczema have a deficien-

cy of the enzyme delta-6 desaturase and as a result produce too little dihomogammalinolenic acid and arachidonic acid. This leads to a deficiency of the prostaglandins which are specifically involved in the prevention of allergic reactions. GLA supplements (such as evening primrose oil) compensate for this deficiency and help in the prevention and treatment of atopic eczema and other allergies.

- Essential fatty acids are vital for the skin, nails and hair. Anyone who suffers from a skin disease such as acne, eczema, dermatitis, psoriasis or sun damage must take supplements of omega-3 and omega-6 fatty acids.

- Essential fatty acids are important for all inflammatory conditions such as all forms of arthritis, muscular injury or myositis and joint pain (arthralgia). The fatty acids helps in the maintenance of the function of the muscles and skeleton. They help prevent osteoporosis. All people who participate in any sport should take supplements of essential fatty acids to improve exercise tolerance, endurance, stamina and performance.

- Essential fatty acids are also used in the treatment of diabetes. Prostaglandins regulate the secretion of insulin by the pancreas, a major problem in diabetes. Research has shown that supplements of essential fatty acids improve the neuropathy often associated with diabetes.

- Essential fatty acids help in the prevention of the severe loss of body weight (cachexia) associated with cancer, AIDS and other debilitating chronic infections such as tuberculosis.

- Essential fatty acids can also help overweight people to loose weight by increasing cell metabolism and allowing the electrolyte and water balance to function in optimal conditions.

- Essential fatty acids are often prescribed for the relief of symptoms associated with premenstrual tension, menopause and other complaints connected with the female urogenital system. They improve fibroadenosis and premenstrual fluid retention.

- The essential fatty acids protect the liver from the toxic effects of alcohol and other poisons.

Essential fatty acids will not necessarily cure all ailments. However, they certainly reduce symptoms and prevent further complications. They restore tissue function at an almost imperceptible and very subtle level. It is not surprising that essential fatty acids are recommended as a vital part of every person's daily food supplement routine.

10 The role of calcium and magnesium

In recent years the Institute of Medicine of the Food and Drug Administration in the United States (FDA) has reconsidered the scientific literature on calcium, phosphorus, magnesium, vitamin D and fluoride metabolism in humans and re-analysed it. They released their findings in August 1997 in an attempt to establish new guidelines for minimum, adequate and maximum daily requirements. The report on calcium et al. was completed first and this is the only group of micronutrients for which the recommended daily allowance (RDA) is really accurate and up to date.

Calcium

The requirement for **calcium** is between 1 000 mg and 1 300 mg a day. The chief source of calcium is dairy products. Calcium is also found in reasonable quantities in leafy green vegetables, egg yolk, pulses (legumes) and nuts. It is almost impossible to obtain enough calcium for normal daily requirements through food alone. Everyone should take supplements: 600 mg per day for general needs, and menopausal and postmenopausal women should take 900-1 000 mg a day. All those who participate in sport should take at least 600 mg of calcium and 300 mg of magnesium a day. This will improve their endurance and performance (by improving heart and lung function), prevent muscular and bone injuries and ensure that muscles, ligaments and bones that are injured, heal more quickly.

Osteoporosis

Calcium is best known for its role in strengthening bone for the prevention and treatment of **osteoporosis**. Apart from calcium intake, other factors are also involved in bone density and the ability of bone to retain calcium. These factors include the growth rate of children at certain stages of their development (for example during the teenager years, where young girls especially tend to cut down on dairy products for fear of putting on weight), hormone status (lower oestrogen levels after menopause result in less calcium being stored in bone), exercise (low impact exercise such as walking improves bone density), genetic heredity (osteoporosis tends to occur in families) and other factors to do with lifestyle (high alcohol intake and smoking accelerate the onset of osteoporosis). Long-term stress leads to increased cortisol levels, which in turn lead to an increased risk for developing osteoporosis.

Osteoporosis is a slow-developing, dormant disease where bone density diminishes and the bones become increasingly brittle and crumble easily. The average loss of bone density in women over 35 is 0,5-1,0 per cent a year. Although all people develop osteoporosis, its severity differs among individuals and between men and women. Women develop osteoporosis earlier than men because the oestrogen that promotes calcium deposits in the bone, decreases markedly around menopause. In men testosterone levels decline more gradually; thus osteoporosis in men develops more slowly. Not all women get osteoporosis to the same extent; a genetic tendency to serious osteoporosis occurs in families. Smoking, low calcium intake, excessive alcohol intake and lack of exercise over a lifetime can play an important role. Slight women often have a fine bone structure with a low calcium content and are thus more prone to develop osteoporosis.

A major problem in osteoporosis is that bones break easily, especially the vertebrae (causing the collapse of the spine, compression of the discs between the vertebrae, severe pain and nerve symptoms) and the head of the femur in the hip joint. If the bone breaks, it is so thin that it takes a long time to knit. Osteoporosis can thus be the cause of an elderly person with an active, healthy, purposeful lifestyle ending up permanently in a wheelchair or bedridden, totally dependent on the support of others for even the most basic functions. This often leads to severe depression and unhappiness. **Osteoporosis can be prevented** by taking calcium supplements from an early age. It is never too late to start taking calcium. Calcium is needed for so many bodily functions that if the body does not have enough for its needs, it simply takes calcium from the bone. Calcium supplements therefore prevent the osteoporosis from becoming worse. Research has also shown that, even if oestrogen and testosterone levels are low, the calcium is still deposited in the bone. In such a case the osteoporosis may even improve with the use of supplemental calcium.

Phosphorus and fluoride

Phosphorus is an important nutrient for the growth and development of bone and soft tissue. It is plentiful in so many types of food that only advanced starvation or a metabolic disorder will result in a lack of phosphorus in the body. It is thus unnecessary to supplement it.

Fluoride is a very controversial topic today. Many research papers indicate that fluoride in drinking water and toothpaste leads to an increased risk of developing cancer, hip fractures (osteoporosis), fluorosis (mottling of the teeth) and liver damage – and does not reduce tooth decay at all. After 50 years of fluoride promotion, it now seems to have been an enormous scam based on misinformation and greed. People are also unhappy about adding fluoride to drinking water because there is no control on the amount of fluoride they are taking in. People who drink a lot of water and babies and children consume far too much fluoride. The FDA in the United States does not regard fluoride as an essential micronutrient.

Magnesium

Magnesium works in conjunction with many of the enzymes in the body to maintain body temperature, nerve conduction, hormone activity, muscle contraction (including the function of the cardiac muscle) and synthesis of proteins. Magnesium is involved in more than 300 different enzyme reactions. The metabolism of calcium and magnesium and their mutual functions are also interdependent. Magnesium is mainly an intracellular mineral (within the cells). Most of the calcium and magnesium (about 70-80 per cent) is stored in the skeleton (bone). A total of 20-30 per cent of the body's magnesium is in the muscles and only 2 per cent is outside the cells, for example in the blood. Magnesium levels in the blood are thus not a good indication of magnesium levels in the body.

Research has shown that hypertension and diabetes are linked to low levels of magnesium in the cells, but it has not yet been established whether the low magnesium is the cause or the effect. However, magnesium levels appear to be a better indicator of these diseases than calcium or sodium.

Low magnesium levels can result in slow digestion of food and increased irritability, along with tremor, muscle spasm, muscle cramps, muscle strain and facial tics. In severe cases this can lead to convulsions, confusion, hallucination, weakness, anorexia, nausea and vomiting. These symptoms are not only caused by a lack of magnesium. This is why it is so difficult to detect a magnesium deficiency.

People who have **blood pressure problems** and **diabetics** should supplement their diet with about 300 mg of magnesium. Some nutritionists are of the opinion that the normal diet can supply enough magnesium for the average person. Magnesium is found in dairy products, vegetables, fish and poultry. Other good sources of magnesium are soya bean flour, wheatgerm, bran, sesame seeds, peanuts and cocoa beans. (Note that cravings for chocolate can be due to a lack of magnesium.)

The main problem with magnesium is that only 30-50 per cent of the daily intake is absorbed. Any additional calcium intake also interferes with the absorption of magnesium. Vitamin D, proteins and lactose promote the absorption of magnesium (and calcium). **If a person is taking a calcium supplement, it is thus essential to take magnesium with it. You must take calcium; so also take 300-500 mg of magnesium together with vitamin D.**

Calcium and magnesium compete for absorption in the digestive tract of the body; so the ratio between the two has to be optimally balanced. Based on the recommended daily allowance, the ratio of calcium to magnesium should be about two to one. This ratio can be used as a general indicator for food supplementation. People who take magnesium supplements must also take calcium.

People who take too many laxatives may take in too much magnesium. Most laxatives contain a large amount of magnesium. Side effects can include low blood pressure, weakness and exhaustion. Elderly people with weakened kidney function can display these side effects even after a few days of injudicious laxative intake. (Milk of magnesia is one of the worst offenders in this respect.)

The role of vitamins D, C and boron

The body gets most of its **vitamin D** from sunlight. As long as people get enough exposure to the sun, it is not necessary to supplement this. However, it is a good idea to take vitamin D with calcium and magnesium for balance and the optimal absorption of both these important micronutrients. Vitamin D improves the bioavailability of calcium. Take 200-400 IU of vitamin D with your calcium and magnesium every evening.

Vitamin C ensures that the calcium is absorbed into the osteoblasts. These are the bone cells that are responsible for the formation of bone and the deposits of calcium in the bone. It is thus also advisable to take about 200 mg of vitamin C in the evenings with your calcium and magnesium. Vitamin C also plays a role in the relief of backache, pain caused by slipped discs and all inflammatory pain associated with arthritis and exercise-induced muscular and joint injuries.

Boron (2 mg a day) is important for the metabolism of calcium, magnesium and phosphorus. It can be used in the treatment of arthritis and hypertension because of its effect on the metabolism of calcium and magnesium. Boron can also prevent the removal of calcium from the bone.

A lot of research has shown that calcium supplementation, especially with magnesium included, plays no role in the formation of calcium oxalate stones in the kidney. High sodium intake (as found in table salt) plays a greater role in the formation of calcium oxalate stones than calcium. Magnesium is often used to treat oxalate stones. Vitamin C plays no role in the development and growth of kidney stones.

Form of intake and bonding of minerals

The suffix -oxalate brings us to the next important point, namely the form in which minerals such as calcium should be taken. A mineral has to be bonded before it can be absorbed from the digestive tract. If minerals are bonded with salts such as carbonates, sulphates and oxides, the mineral salt compounds have to go through a long, complicated digestive and absorption process before they can be absorbed by the body. This process can lead to constipation, nausea, black stools (such as caused by iron-mineral salt compounds taken during pregnancy) and bloating.

The best way of bonding is a chelation process in which minerals are linked to amino acids. Amino acid bonding is also the natural way in which the body absorbs minerals and transports them through the walls of the intestine. Amino acids are the building blocks of proteins and are thus natural products which the body recognises as such.

By bonding minerals to amino acids, excellent absorption, bioavailability (optimal utilisation of minerals by the body) and biological activity of minerals in the body is assured. The safety and tolerance of the body to such minerals are also excellent and side effects are rare. The amino acid-mineral compound is absorbed as a whole. In the liver the amino acids are metabolised further and the minerals are released into the blood to perform all their necessary functions. These amino acids must be in the stomach and the rest of the digestive tract at the same time as the minerals so that chelation can occur.

Try to buy mineral supplements that are already in an amino acid chelation. However, the manufacturing process of amino acid chelates of high quality is expensive. When choosing a mineral supplement, you get what you pay for. If you can't find a calcium product in an amino acid chelation or if it is too expensive, the next best way to take in calcium is as a carbonate, gluconate or lactate. Food form minerals are also well absorbed by the body. Food form is, as the name implies, extracts from food complexes

Calcium and magnesium supplements

Some calcium and magnesium supplements may also contain:

- **Potassium** (about 200 mg per day) is important for the correct pH-balance of the metabolism of calcium and magnesium in bones and muscles (cardiac, skeletal and smooth muscle). Potassium stabilises the internal structure of cells and is essential for nervous, cardiac and musculoskeletal function. Potassium is generally used for the treatment of hypertension, exhaustion and muscular weakness. It is also useful for treating allergies.
- **Glycine** (about 250 mg a day) is an amino acid which is an excellent natural sedative.

Remember to take calcium and magnesium supplements at night. This ensures that the nervous system is less irritable and allows the musculoskeletal system to relax. Causes of insomnia include being unable to switch off one's thoughts, having a continuous 'monkey chatter' in your mind and not being able to relax.

Calcium, magnesium and glycine help to calm down the thought processes (in addition to relaxation techniques and meditation). Glycine has been used successfully to treat spastic conditions of the nervous system, anxiety attacks, to improve wound healing and epilepsy. Glycine is an important component of collagen which forms part of the connective tissue in bone, cartilage, joints and muscle. Glycine reduces acidity in the stomach and is useful in the treatment of ulcers, gastritis, reflux and heartburn. Glycine also delays the degeneration of muscle tissue by providing additional creatinine. Creatinine is present in all muscles and is essential for muscle contraction and relaxation. Glycine and creatinine are involved in the formation of RNA and DNA (nuclear matter). Glycine is also essential in the synthesis of haemoglobin (the molecules that carry the oxygen in the red blood cells) and glutathione (an important part of the antioxidant enzyme glutathione peroxidase).

- **L-taurine** (about 250 mg a day) is an amino acid with various functions. (Consult Chapter 7 on the cardiovascular system.) Taurine is important for the relaxation of the muscles after contraction. It preserves antioxidants and stabilises cell membranes. It facilitates the movement of potassium, sodium, magnesium and calcium across the cell membranes. It is thus important for the generation and conduction of nerve impulses. Taurine is often used with magnesium in treating epilepsy, anxiety, tension, high cholesterol, hypertension, arrhythmia (irregular heartbeat) and insomnia.
- **Methyl sulphonyl methane** (MSM, about 200 mg a day) is a natural, safe physiological active sulphur compound with anti-inflammatory and antioxidant properties. It is also used for the treatment of all forms of arthritis and joint infection. It supplies sulphur for the formation of healthy connective tissue, enzymes and compounds which are effective in fighting allergies. MSM strengthens the body's natural defence against allergens (substances that induce an allergic reaction in sensitive people). Sulphur is also essential for healthy hair, skin and nails. MSM fights parasites, improves general digestion and helps to relax tense, tired muscles and joints. People who suffer from allergies often have a lack of calcium. Calcium supplements with MSM alleviate most forms of allergy.
- **Phytosterols** (about 50-100 mg a day) are natural substances that are present in all plants (also called plant sterols). They are also the part of the plant that is often removed through food processing (wheatgerm is rich in phytosterols). Phytosterols are built into the cell membrane as part of the phospholipid chain and improve the transfer of calcium through the cell membrane into the cell. They therefore improve the bioavailability of calcium.
- **Silica** (about 20 mg a day) stimulates the cells that are responsible for the formation of collagen and elastin, the connective tissue that is found in the bone matrix and beneath the skin. It prevents the skin from losing its elasticity and the loss of bone density. Silica improves

the elasticity of blood vessels and plays an important role in the pre-vention of cardiovascular diseases. It is also important in preventing osteoporosis and Alzheimer's disease. It strengthens the immune function and delays the ageing process of tissue.

- **Manganese** (about 20 mg a day) nourishes the nervous system and improves sugar and fat metabolism. It is essential for the formation of DNA and RNA and prevents fatigue, irritability and sensitivity of the nervous system, as well as lower back pain. It reduces the frequency of epileptic seizures. Manganese forms part of the antioxidant enzyme superoxide dismutase, which protects the body from the damage by free radicals. Manganese improves the immune function and prevents atherosclerosis, poor hair and nail growth, hearing loss and poor muscle and joint co-ordination.
- **Copper** (about 2-4 mg a day) is important in the formation of bone, haemoglobin and red blood cells. It works in conjunction with vitamin C, zinc and silica to form elastin. Copper helps to control the inflammatory reaction in arthritis and bursitis. It is important for a healthy nervous system and smooth joint operation. Copper also helps with the mineralisation of bone (calcium deposits) and is also part of many antioxidant enzyme systems.

Summary of the functions of calcium and magnesium

- Calcium and magnesium are important in the prevention and treatment of osteoporosis.
- Both calcium and magnesium are extremely effective natural sedatives (for insomnia and tension or anxiety). Always take them at bedtime with a hot drink. This is also good for children who sleep badly or are hyperactive.
- Calcium and magnesium ensure healthy hair, bone growth, teeth and strong nails – especially important for children and people whose nails and hair are brittle and break easily. Increase your intake after any bone fracture.
- Supplementation is essential for pregnant women and women who are breastfeeding – for the mother's needs as well as those of the unborn foetus and growing baby. Supplement with 600 mg of calcium and 300 mg of magnesium a day. If your intake of dairy products is low (or absent), use 900 mg of calcium and 450 mg of magnesium.

- Calcium and magnesium are essential in the treatment of hypertension and other disorders of the cardiovascular system.
- Most cases of headache will be cured by taking 300-600 mg of calcium and 150-300 mg of magnesium instead of a headache pill. It is also an effective treatment for migraine. It is worth trying.
- Remember that calcium and magnesium can be used for all forms of allergy. Children and adults who are allergic to dairy products in any case take in too little calcium and magnesium in their diet.
- All those who participate in sport should take calsium and magnesium supplements to be able to cope with the increased demands made on the body's metabolism, enzymes, and musculoskeletal system.
- Calcium and magnesium provide great relief from all forms of leg cramps (also night cramps) and growing pains in children.
- Calcium and magnesium alleviate the symptoms of premenstrual tension (depression, irritability, headaches, moodiness, bloating, backache and cramps), menopause and painful menstruation.
- Calcium and magnesium can also reduce the symptoms of tinnitus (ringing in the ears) and vertigo (dizziness when moving).
- Calcium and magnesium can help to alleviate the symptoms of multiple sclerosis and other forms of muscular dystrophy because of its important function in muscle contraction.
- Calcium and magnesium improve neural transfer and are recommended in the treatment of depression, hyperactivity and anxiety conditions.
- Calcium and magnesium are essential in the treatment of low blood sugar levels as well as in diabetes (people with high blood sugar levels).
- Research shows that calcium plays a major role in the prevention and treatment of cancer (especially of the colon and rectum).

11 Micronutrients for the musculoskeletal system

The micronutrients involved here ensure that the muscles and skeletal frame function optimally. They provide support in case of any disorder of the muscles, joints, ligaments and bones in the body. Examples of these diseases are arthritis (osteoarthritis, gout and rheumatoid arthritis), myositis (infection of the muscles), myalgia (muscular pain), arthralgia (pain in the joints), osteoporosis, inflammation of the joints and muscles (fibrositis) and all forms of muscle injury.

Inflammation is the normal reaction of the body after infection and injury. It is a healing reaction. The redness, swelling, pain and heat that are characteristic of an inflammatory reaction prove that the body's nervous, vascular, immune and hormone systems are activated and accelerating the body's resistance and recovery. Illness occurs when inflammation goes on for too long and no longer serves its purpose. Chronic inflammation is a problem in almost all diseases of the musculoskeletal system, as well as with autoimmune diseases.

Inflammation is usually treated with corticosteroids (metabolic disorders can be a problem – corticosteroids are toxic and immunosuppressive in the long term) and anti-inflammatory medications (which can damage the mucosa of the stomach and suppress the immune system). Natural alternatives are more effective and less harmful – in most cases not harmful at all.

Conventional treatment of all forms of arthritis and other inflammatory conditions is palliative – the condition is alleviated but not cured. However, research has shown that changes in diet and lifestyle with stress management and supplementation can favourably influence the disease process. Arthritis is a metabolic disorder that occurs after a lifetime of stress (physical, chemical and emotional), incorrect eating habits, too little exercise and a negative attitude to life. These stress factors negatively influence glandular secretion (hormones), digestion of food and the utilisation and excretion of nutrients. This leads to suppression of the immune system, the development of allergies and eventually to inflammatory diseases such as arthritis.

A diet low in saturated fats, mainly vegetarian, combined with stress management, exercise and correct supplementation can really get to the root of the problem. Food supplements have brought about remarkable improvements in about 80-90 per cent of arthritis sufferers.

Backache is another common problem that is seldom healed by using conventional medication. Remember that therapeutic massage with essential oils (lavender, thyme, eucalyptus, pine and juniper berry) and realignment of the body by the application of kinesiology and chiropractic can be of great value in treating backache and other inflammatory processes. Lifestyle adaptations, stress management, supplementation and exercise are of inestimable value in treating the cause of the problem.

Inflammation is regulated by prostaglandins (consult Chapter 9). Some strengthen the anti-inflammatory reaction while others suppress it.

Micronutrients for optimal functioning

1 Essential fatty acids

Gamma linolenic acid (omega-6) leads to the formation of prostaglandins that suppress the inflammatory process. Alpha linolenic acid, eicosapentaenoic and docosahexanoic acid (omega-3) lead to the suppression of the inflammatory reaction. Use them for at least six to 12 weeks before expecting results. (Consult chapter 9.)

2 Calcium, magnesium et al.

All these ingredients are essential for the treatment of all disorders of the musculoskeletal system and maintaining it in peak condition. (Consult Chapter 10 for more information.)

3 Multivitamin, antioxidant and mineral combinations

Quantities given here are higher because a disorder in the relevant system already exists. These should contain all the usual ingredients, with the emphasis on the following:

● **Vitamin A** (10 000 IU a day or 3 030 micrograms or 3 mg of vitamin A or RE activity) is involved in depositing new bone. Vitamin A accelerates the repair and healing of damaged tissue (after infection, muscle strain and surgery) and prevents infection. Vitamin A also protects all tissue linings (including the synovial membranes in the joints, the periosteum which covers the long bones, and cartilage) from damage by free radicals.

- **Vitamin E** (400 IU or 332 mg a day) reduces chronic inflammatory damage to tissue (such as inflammation in arthritic joints) by restricting the damage by free radicals. Free radicals can considerably harm already infected joints; they lead to the formation of more free radicals in a vicious circle. Vitamin E delays the degeneration and ageing of tissue and is used in the treatment of muscle cramps, injured muscles, osteoarthritis, autoimmune diseases (rheumatoid arthritis and arthritis associated with psoriasis) and infections.

- **Vitamin C** (500-1 000 mg twice a day) plays an important role in the formation and maintenance of collagen, the main ingredient of all connective tissue. Connective tissue is responsible for the support and shape of the skin, ligaments, cartilage, intervertebral discs, synovium (joint linings), bones and teeth. Vitamin C is commonly used in treating arthritis, sports injuries, overtraining and bursitis. Vitamin C also has antioxidant and anti-inflammatory properties and is vital for the deposit of calcium into the osteoblasts (bone-forming cells) to prevent osteoporosis.

- All the **B-complex vitamins** are important for the functioning of the musculoskeletal system. Vitamin B2 (50 mg a day) is used to treat leg cramps. Vitamin B3 (50 mg a day) is used in the treatment of arthritis to assist in improving blood flow. It also improves blood circulation in the legs and can help in cases where the blood flow has been reduced (e.g. winter hands and feet, Raynaud's syndrome, diabetic arterial insufficiency). Vitamin B5 (50 mg a day) has an anti-inflammatory effect. Vitamin B6 (50-100 mg a day) is used to treat muscular pain, tired muscles, neuritis and carpal tunnel syndrome. Folic acid (400 micrograms a day) is used for restless leg syndrome, neuropathy, gout and osteoporosis.

- **Copper** (4 mg a day) helps vitamin C in the formation of collagen and connective tissue. It accelerates the healing of tissue and improves suppleness of the ligaments. It has been used for centuries for the treatment of arthritis and other inflammatory conditions.

- **Manganese** (5 mg a day) is important for the normal growth of bone. Vitamin C and manganese increase the effectiveness of chondroitin and glucosamine (see page 138).

- **Zinc** (15 mg a day) is important in protein synthesis and collagen formation. (Consult Chapter 5 on antioxidants.)

4 Medicinal herbs

- **Ginger** is a well-known anti-inflammatory herbal cure. Drink it as a tea or use it as part of a herbal mixture with standardised extracts of **turmeric** (curcuminoids have an anti-inflammatory effect), **fever-few** (anti-inflammatory and analgesic), ***Boswellia serrata*, kava kava** and/or **white willow bark** (*Salix alba*, natural aspirin that does not harm the mucosa of the stomach).
- **Bromelain**, an enzyme found in the stem of the pineapple (*Ananas sativus*), can be used in standardised extract form to alleviate all inflammatory processes. It is especially valuable in the treatment of arthritis, sports injuries and to reduce postoperative swelling.

(Consult Chapters 5 and 6 – the medicinal herbs as antioxidants and discussed for participation in sport will also help to reduce the considerable damage caused by free radicals associated with arthritis and other inflammatory diseases.)

5 Amino acids
(500-1 000 mg a day on an empty stomach with 500 mg of vitamin C, 50-100 mg of vitamin B6 and 400 micrograms of folic acid)

- **L-histidine** levels are often lower in people with arthritis (especially rheumatoid arthritis). Research has shown that histidine supplements improve the strength and mobility of arthritis sufferers. Histidine also has potent anti-inflammatory properties.
- **L-proline** is abundant in the collagen structure of the synovia (joint membranes) and improves the mobility of joints in arthritis sufferers and after sports injuries.
- **DL-phenyl alanine** is an amino acid that research has shown to be effective in the treatment of chronic pain. It raises the levels of the endorphins, the brain's own analgesic or painkilling hormones. It is used to treat backache and arthritis. If you suffer from phenylketonuria, however, or are taking a monoamino oxidase inhibitor for depression, you should not take it without the supervision and approval of your doctor or health care provider.

- **Glucosamine sulphate** (1 000 mg a day) is an amino acid-glucose compound which occurs naturally in cartilage. It functions as supportive building material and stimulates the production of other ingredients that are essential for the functioning of the cartilage and joints. Clinical studies have shown that glucosamine sulphate supplements are effective in the long-term treatment of arthritis. There are no known side effects or contraindications for its use. Glucosamine improves the inflammatory reaction and research has shown conclusively that glucosamine sulphate considerably alleviates painful joints, tenderness and swelling. There is also a marked improvement in the mobility of the joints in arthritis sufferers. In some studies there was even a reversal of the cartilage degeneration. In several European countries glucosamine sulphate is the first line of treatment for arthritis, taking precedence over conventional medicines.
- **Chondroitin** improves the fluid content of the cartilage and joints and in this way improves the supply of glucose and nutrients to the joints. It also improves the shock-absorbent function of the cartilage. Chondroitin sulphate is manufactured from the cartilage of cattle, sharks and whales. If you have ethical objections to using animal products, glucosamine sulphate on its own is just as effective.

Glucosamine sulphate and chondroitin sulphate work in conjunction to protect the cartilage from degeneration (degradation, waste and attenuation so that the bones forming joints begin to rub against each other). Both provide the raw material for the formation of new cartilage. Glucosamine sulphate, chondroitin sulphate, vitamin C and manganese work in synergy to strengthen your body's own natural healing mechanisms.

Case study

As an example of a holistic approach to a chronic inflammatory condition, let me describe my own path to recovery after acute and chronic back problems.

Our family has a history of back problems. In my case, whenever there are lifestyle difficulties and long-term stress, the musculoskeletal system collapses first.

In March 1997 I damaged my back while playing squash. I was unfit and launched myself into the game without warming up properly. At least twice a year before this incident I would battle with a bad back, which usually calmed down after a few days. This time the injury was much worse. I took painkillers and anti-inflammatories and hoped for the best. Unfortunately, I largely ignored the back problem at that stage and struggled along with a shortened right leg that compensated for the muscle spasm in the back.

In September 1997 the pain returned – this time acutely. My right leg and foot went lame and there was no feeling in my lower back and buttocks. This frightened me because I realised that the nerve root was damaged. This usually indicates a serious problem. X-rays showed that the fifth lumbar vertebra had slipped backwards onto the first sacral vertebra, placing the spinal cord and nerves under tension. This was causing the acute pain and lack of sensation.

Conventional medicine offers very few solutions for backache: painkillers, anti-inflammatories, in some cases corticosteroids, physiotherapy, a few exercises and then the only answer is major surgery such as spinal fusion, with a success rate of 50-60 per cent. I began to panic. The first few options were not successful. The pain was so bad that I took to my bed and my muscles began to atrophy. (Muscles get weak very quickly when they are not used.) My interest in alternative healing made me distrustful of surgery – it went against my philosophy of holistic and gentle healing.

The greatest single factor that put me on the road to recovery was the day I took control of my state of mind and emotions. Mental and emotional control are an important part of any chronic disease, be it pain or cancer. Fear and panic are the most harmful factors that send all disease processes into a downward spiral and make them worse.

The following measures have systematically solved the problem to a great extent:

- The awareness and recognition that stress played a major role in my back problem. Moving to Somerset West after a financial disaster in Pretoria, worrying about the children adjusting to a new environment, starting a new practice, my new magazine and at the same time my first book (published and marketed on my own), plans for the new house and all the financial implications associated with that, had started to take their toll after about two years. This was the first time I had experienced at first hand the effects of long-term stress on my own health. Financial tension will manifest in the first energy chakra with lower back problems. I began to apply relaxation techniques such as progressive muscle relaxation and meditation.

Visualisation techniques in which I sometimes pictured myself dancing around and at other times placed myself in a peaceful rustic
scene reinforced the message of healing. The whole process taught
me a lot and helped me in my treatment of patients with chronic diseases. Once the period of denial and suppression of negative emotions has passed, the healing process can begin.

- A diet consisting of lots of fresh fruit and vegetables, with wholegrain
products and fish, alleviated the chronic constipation associated with
the nerve compression and prevented me from putting on weight
from all the inactivity. The following Ayurvedic recipe (and grand-
ma's!) finally sorted out my severe constipation: 1 tablespoon of cas-
tor oil before bedtime in a quarter of a glass of hot water containing
a pinch of ginger and a few drops of lemon juice (it also takes away
the oily taste). Drink this for one or two evenings and then again
after a week. You should not do this more than once a month.

- Correct supplements to restore the functioning of the musculoskeletal and nervous systems included the following:
  – Calcium, magnesium, vitamins D and C, B-complex, potassium,
  zinc, copper, boron, silica and manganese.
  – Essential fatty acids (gamma linolenic, eicosapentanoic and
  docosahexanoic acids in the form of evening primrose oil capsules
  (2 000 mg a day) and salmon oil capsules (1 200 mg a day).
  – Antioxidants with vitamins A, E and C as well as selenium and the
  herbs cat's claw (Uncaria tomentosa), Pycnogenol, ginger, turmeric,
  white willow bark, kava kava and pineapple extract with bromelain.

- Deep therapeutic back massage, reflexology and chiropractic, as well
as Maitland therapy, acupressure (a form of acupuncture) and ultrasound therapy by a qualified physiotherapist, a therapeutic masseuse
and a careful, gentle chiropractor improved the muscle spasm and
the misaligned vertebrae. The chiropractor eased the vertebrae back
into position with corrective manipulation. Essential oils such as
lavender, eucalyptus, thyme, pine and camomile were used for the
massaging. Add them to your bathwater to promote relaxation of the
muscles and generally help you to unwind.

- The correct exercises for the tummy muscles, upper thighs and buttocks gradually strengthened the back muscles to support the vertebrae better. I also started walking regularly.

I will always have to be careful. Even after months of regular exercise,
correct eating and stress management, it is easy to forget your good

habits – in as little as two weeks. Lifestyle adaptations are obviously required, but it is not easy to change habits and make them a permanent part of your life. Be patient and keep at it!

Note: It is essential for conventional doctors and complementary health care providers to work together to the benefit of all parties, especially with the ailing and unhealthy state of humankind as it is today. My back problem is a good example of the many health problems where different therapeutic disciplines can support one another and work together to ensure optimal health and wellbeing.

12 Micronutrients for the nervous system

All the organs are important for the balanced functioning of body and soul. The brain can be considered the chief conductor of the orchestra of the body, intellect and mind. The brain controls an amazing number of functions. The best computer in the world does not even have one hundredth of the capacity of the human brain. The brain is responsible for every biochemical and physiological function, for every emotion and thought, from the most basic urges to our highest thoughts and ideals. It is also the organ that brings us as close as possible to our soul. The nervous system, endocrine system (hormonal system) and immune system are inseparably linked to one another and any disorder in one system often leads to disorder in the other two. (Consult Chapters 1 and 2 on stress and its treatment.)

Scientists have tried for many years to unravel the mysteries of the brain. This process of discovery has established that the complicated functions of the brain depend on various nutrients, which have to be in balance. Research is showing increasingly that deficiencies of certain micronutrients and chemical imbalances can affect our emotional, physical and psychological wellbeing.

The brain is metabolically very active. This results in the large-scale production of free radicals. The build-up of free radicals over the years plays an important role in the development of many diseases of the nervous system. Free radicals have an affinity for the lipid (fatty) membranes of the neurons (nerve cells) in the brain. This causes oxidation of the neuron membranes through a process called lipid peroxidation - the common final pathway for the onset of many neurological diseases. Examples include Alzheimer's and Parkinson's disease. Free radicals as metabolic waste from the stress reaction, toxins and infection are also inclined to bond with the lipid membranes of the neurons.

One of the first signs of deterioration in brain function is memory loss. Many elderly people become aware that their memory is failing and immediately decide that they have Alzheimer's disease. This loss of memory can probably be ascribed to high concentrations of free radicals and micronutrient deficiencies, as well as unresolved emotional stress.

Memory loss causes much anxiety and panic. The fear is often a greater problem than the failing memory. Many of us spend our lives madly rushing around in different directions chasing after material things and we seldom focus and concentrate on the moment. If your thoughts are fixed on something from the past or in the future, you are quite likely to forget something that you should remember in the present. The motivation to concentrate and remember often disappears as you get older. Learn to live in the moment, follow the guidelines for a healthy lifestyle, exercise, use your supplements and keep your mind active. This is the recipe for eternal youth. If your mind and spirit remain young, active and positive, your body will follow. Over the years you will come to realize that the external condition of the body is far less important than the internal condition of the mind and emotions.

All those who are coping with stress, tension, anxiety, depression, poor memory, poor concentration, Alzheimer's or Parkinson's disease, headaches (where physical causes have been eliminated), attention deficit, tinnitus (ringing in the ears) or vertigo (dizziness) should at least try food supplementation. The success rate is high. Don't forget the importance of exercise for health and the relief of depression, anxiety and tension. Add to this your stress management (including meditation, which can be of great value), the unravelling of all the negativity that has built up, as well as the suppressed emotions and you can expect an improvement or even recovery.

Micronutrients for optimal functioning of the nervous system

1 Antioxidant, multivitamin and mineral combination

Antioxidants are probably one of the best ways to restrict the damage caused by free radicals and allowing the body's own antioxidant enzymes to function optimally. (Consult Chapter 5 on antioxidants.) Make sure that your choice includes the following:

● Vitamin C (500 mg two or three times a day) is an important antioxidant that enhances the function of the antioxidant enzyme glutathione peroxidation. It is also involved in the conversion of tryptophan to hydroxytryptophan which in turn is a precursor of serotonin, an important neurotransmitter that determines our state of mind and emotions. Serotonin is also important for our sleep pattern. Vitamin C also helps in the conversion of tyrosine to the neurotransmitters dopamine, adrenalin and noradrenaline. Adrenalin and noradrenaline are the stress hormones that are secreted during the stress reaction. Extended periods of stress exhaust the body's supply of vitamin C and result in poor management of stress with the development of a negative stress phase. (Consult Chapters 1 and 2.)

- Vitamin A (10 000 IU or 3 030 micrograms or 3 mg of RE or vitamin A activity a day) with beta carotenes and other carotenes (25 000 IU or 15 mg a day) are important for neutralising free radicals after a stroke and for managing vision problems (especially night blindness). Vitamin A is important in restricting the affected area after a stroke. The build-up of free radicals during the stroke can cause the surrounding brain tissue to be affected and the area of nerve loss to increase.
- Vitamin E and other tocopherols (400 IU a day) are fat-soluble antioxidants that prevent damage from the free radicals present in the lipid membrane of the neurons. They are important in the management of stroke, Alzheimer's and Parkinson's disease. Vitamin E also boosts the body's own antioxidant glutathione peroxidation enzyme action.
- Other important antioxidants for the nervous system are green tea, cat's claw, pycnogenol, N-acetyl-L-cysteine, zinc and copper. The last two, together with manganese are important for the functioning of the antioxidant enzyme superoxide dismutase. Pycnogenol (proanthocyanidin), found in grape seeds and pine bark, penetrates the blood-brain barrier and then comes into direct contact with the brain tissue to neutralise free radicals.
- All the B-complex vitamins are essential for the functioning of the nervous system. They are all involved in maintaining the structure and operation of the myelin sheath so that messages can be transmitted effectively. They also perform many other functions. The myelin sheath works exactly like the insulation material around a piece of electric flex.

  If the covering is worn and you touch the wire, you will short-circuit the electric current and get a shock. The electricity no longer follows the effective path. Deterioration of the myelin sheath is one of the main causes of multiple sclerosis. Messages are not transmitted effectively in one direction, but get lost along the 'short-circuited' sections. The same happens to a lesser extent in memory loss, concentration problems and attention deficit disorder.

The B-complex vitamins improve the sleep pattern (for insomnia) and increase the body's ability to handle stress. All the B vitamins work best if they are used with **zinc and magnesium.**

- Vitamin B1 (thiamine, 50 mg a day) facilitates the conversion of glucose into energy as fuel for the brain. It also imitates the neurotransmitter acetylcholine, which is important for memory, perception and knowledge (the cognitive functions). Supplementation with B1 can also improve the state of mind. It is used in the treatment of fatigue, irritability, negative attitude, stress, muscle spasm, multiple sclerosis, neuritis and depression.
- Vitamins B2 and B3 (niacin and riboflavin, 50 mg of each a day) improve neuron transfer and the ability of the body to handle stress. B3 is often used in the treatment of fatigue, irritability, migraine, trigeminal neuralgia, depression and Méunière's disease (loss of hearing together with vertigo).
- Vitamin B5 (pantothenic acid, 50 mg a day) is also called the anti-stress vitamin. It supports the adrenal gland in the production of cortisone and in this way helps to balance the metabolism in managing the effects of long-term stress. As part of co-enzyme A it is important for the formation of acetylcholine.
- Vitamin B6 (pyridoxine, 100 mg a day) is important for amino acid metabolism. It is responsible for the production of an important neurotransmitter in the brain: gamma amino butyric acid (GABA). B6 is also involved in the formation of other neurotransmitters (noradrenaline, acetylcholine and serotonin). It is prescribed to treat most disorders of the nervous system.
- Vitamin B12 (cobalamin, 50 micrograms a day) is known as the longevity vitamin and is important for the normal activity of the nervous system, especially in elderly people. It is often prescribed in the treatment of nervous system disease.
- Folic acid (400 micrograms a day) is essential for the development of the nervous system before birth. A marginal deficiency of folic acid can contribute to the development of many nervous disorders (including depression, epilepsy, neuropathy, stress and fatigue).
- Choline (100 mg a day) together with inositol forms part of lecithin and as part of acetylcholine it is essential for memory, learning ability and intellectual alertness (cognitive functions). Choline is an amino acid which forms part of the B-complex vitamins.

- Inositol (100 mg a day) is present in cell membranes as phosphatidyl inositol. Serotonin and acetylcholine require phosphatidyl inositol in order to function effectively. Inositol is valuable in all disorders of the nervous system. It also helps for insomnia.

2 Calcium and magnesium

Both calcium and magnesium are important for the transfer of messages in the nervous system. They are also involved in the formation of neurotransmitters. Calcium and magnesium reduce nerve and muscle excitability and are an excellent natural remedy for sleeping problems. Magnesium is the antistress mineral and acts as a natural sedative. Supplementation with calcium and magnesium is indicated in all disorders of the nervous system. Calcium alone, however, should not be given to people with Alzheimer's disease – another reason for supplementing with calcium and magnesium! (Consult Chapter 10 on the role of calcium and magnesium.)

3 Essential fatty acids

Docosahexanoic acid (an omega-3 fatty acid) is the most important structural lipid (fat) in the brain. It directly influences the communication between neurons (nerve transmission). DHA is also a calcium channel blocker in the brain. It is very important in Alzheimer's disease where increased calcium levels in the brain can activate the enzyme that is responsible for the formation of ameloid deposits. These deposits play a key role in the development of Alzheimer's because they interfere with memory and the neuron functions. (Consult Chapter 9 on essential fatty acids.)

DHA is vital for the development of the brain and retina in the foetus. The unborn baby gets all the essential fatty acids through the placenta from the mother.

Research has shown that an imbalance in the ratio of omega-3 to omega-6 fatty acids can lead to depression (too much omega-6; a ratio of 50:1 instead of 3:1 omega-6 to omega-3). Lack of omega-3 and omega-6 also plays an important role in attention deficit disorder, poor memory and concentration problems.

4 Amino acids

Remember to always take amino acids with vitamin C (200-500 mg), vitamin B6 (100 mg) and a little fruit juice for better absorption and efficacy. Choose one or two amino acids to supplement the functioning of the nervous system.

- Phosphatidyl serine (100 mg a day – an expensive supplement) is a combination of the amino acid serine and phospholipids. It occurs naturally in the brain of animals and in soya products. It is the main phospholipid in the brain and forms part of the cell membrane. It therefore plays a major role in the fluidity and integrity of the cell membrane. Phosphatidyl serine (PS) improves intellectual functions even in healthy individuals. As the brain starts to age, the fluidity of the cell membrane diminishes. This causes a rigid, stiff structure that distorts nerve transmission. The messages become tangled in the hardened tissue. In degenerative brain diseases such as Alzheimer's this process occurs at a much younger age. PS supplements improve memory and intellectual alertness (cognitive functions) in young and old. Restored neuron fluidity results in an increase in acetylcholine receptors. PS also helps to prevent the neurons and axons from becoming tangled.

  Research has shown that PS can even reverse existing brain damage. It is recommended for the treatment of senile dementia, Alzheimer's disease, severe stress and mental exhaustion, depression and poor memory. It improves cognitive and behavioural functions in dementia and memory loss.
- DL-phenyl alanine (500 mg a day) is the precursor of dopamine, noradrenaline and adrenaline, the stimulating neurotransmitters. It increases the levels of endorphins which are the natural painkillers in the brain. Endorphins also improve the state of mind. DL-phenyl alanine is recommended for the treatment of depression, chronic mental exhaustion and appetite control. It should not, however, be used by people who suffer from phenylketonuria.
- L-tyrosine (500 mg a day) is a precursor of noradrenaline, adrenalin and dopamin, the neurotransmitters responsible for mental alertness and clarity. Increased levels of these neuronutrients can have a positive effect on attitude and behavioural patterns. Tyrosine is also needed for thyroid hormone synthesis. It is also valuable in treating depression, mental exhaustion, stress-related anxiety and hypothyroidism.

- Acetyl-L-carnitine (250 mg a day) is similar to acetylcholine in structure and has a similar effect on the nervous system. It is also an antioxidant and protects the nervous system from the damage by free radicals. It promotes the synthesis of phospholipids such as phosphatidyl serine and improves brain energy metabolism – the brain's utilisation of glucose for energy. Acetyl-L-carnitine improves memory and mental alertness. It is recommended for senile dementia and Alzheimer's disease.
- L-tryptophan and hydroxytryptophan are the precursors of serotonin, the neurotransmitter that has a calming, antidepressant and sleep-inducing effect. Tryptophan is abundant in bananas, milk and sunflower seeds. Since 1989 it has not been available in supplement form because of possible side effects on the nerves and muscles. It has subsequently been proved that these side effects were caused by bacterial contamination in one of the supply sources. The ban on tryptophan, however, has since been lifted.
- L-taurine (500 mg a day) is a neurotransmitter that has a calming effect on the nervous system. It therefore has a calming influence in the case of attention deficit disorder, anxiety, tension, epilepsy, panic attacks and insomnia. Taurine also protects the eyes from damage because of its antioxidant properties. Zinc enhances the effect of taurine.
- L-glutamine (500 mg a day) is used by the brain and central nervous system together with other amino acids such as choline, tyrosine and phenyl alanine to form neurotransmitters. The neurotransmitters pass messages from one nerve to the next and can stimulate or suppress the electrical impulses in the brain that lead to thoughts, feelings and emotions. Different neurotransmitters also affect our perception of chronic fatigue and dejection, or simply the will to live. Neurotransmitters often become exhausted in the normal functioning of the body. Physical or psychological stress causes the body to metabolise and use more neurotransmitters and supplementation with these important biochemical nutrients is thus essential. Glutamine with vitamin B6 and manganese is a precursor of gamma amino butyric acid (GABA), an important neurotransmitter with a greater suppressant and calming effect. Glutamine also contributes to mental alertness and improved memory. It is used in the treatment of fatigue and anxiety, Parkinsonism, schizophrenia, mental degeneration and muscular dystrophy. Glutamine is a precursor of growth hormone and can help to delay the ageing process.
- Glycine (500 mg a day) is one of the main suppressant neurotrans-

mitters in the brain and is recommended for anxiety, tension and panic attacks. It is also valuable in treating attention deficit disorder.

5 Medicinal herbs

Many herbal remedies are effective for treating disorders of the nervous system and the brain. Our discussion here is thus restricted to a few that have been well researched in the West.

Remember that the adaptogens such as Korean, American and Siberian ginseng, Reishi, Maitaki and Shiitake mushrooms, astragalus and liquorice root are all helpful in protecting the body against the negative effects of long-term stress. (Consult Chapters 1 and 2 on stress and its treatment.) The adaptogens support the adrenal function so that the body is less susceptible to the exhaustion that is associated with chronic stress. Adaptogens play a role in all the systems of the body where the genetic composition of a particular person will result in the expression of negative stress in a specific system. (For example, eczema is a skin manifestation of stress and asthma is a respiratory tract manifestation of stress.) It is usually sufficient to take one adaptogen for stress. Supplements that contain adaptogens are usually obtainable in combinations. Make sure that the product you use is from a reliable and expert source.

Ginkgo (*Ginkgo biloba*, maidenhair tree)
(60 mg twice a day)

Ginkgo is probably the most essential ingredient in a nervous system supplement. As the life expectancy of humans increases, more attention is focused on the different ways of retaining mental alertness and clarity. Even younger people are interested in ways of keeping the mind clear and concentration optimal – it's a good way of maintaining the advantage in a competitive business environment.

Ginkgo extract is made from the leaves of a tree known as *Ginkgo biloba* – the oldest species of tree in the world, a living fossil, indigenous to China. The leaves have the shape of the two lobes of the brain. This is the herb most commonly prescribed by doctors in Germany and France. Throughout the world ginkgo is prescribed for all problems concerned with blood circulation, especially in the brain. It is preferable for ginkgo to be taken in standardised form, containing 24 per cent glycosides and 6 per cent terpene lactones.

A research study published in the journal of the Medical Association of America has shown that ginkgo works much better than a placebo in the treatment of Alzheimer's disease. The side effect profile for this sensitive group of patients was also remarkably low.

Ginkgo improves the blood flow to the brain so that the brain gets more oxygen and glucose. On a cellular level ginkgo stabilises cell membranes, disposes of free radicals, stimulates enzymes that allow the arterial smooth muscle to relax (important in hypertension and stroke) and suppresses platelet aggregation (important in the treatment and prevention of hypertension, heart attacks and stroke).

Ginkgo has two groups of active ingredients: the glycosides which include the bioflavonoids (for example quercetin) and the terpene lactones which include the ginkgolides and bilobalides.

The bioflavonoids promote the antioxidant activity of ginkgo in the brain and cardiovascular system. (Consult Chapters 5 and 7.) They also reduce platelet aggregation.

However, it is the ginkgolides and bilobalides that make ginkgo unique. These are the ingredients that improve the flow of blood to the brain and other parts of the body so that the tissue gets more oxygen, nutrients and glucose for energy. They also protect the neurons throughout the body and are responsible for ginkgo's ability to improve memory and mental function. This is especially important for elderly people who are showing signs of declining cognitive function (the mental process in which knowledge is acquired, including memory and perception). Ginkgolides and bilobalides suppress the platelet activation factor, a substance that can cause nerve damage, poor blood flow to the brain and constriction of the airways in the lungs, all of which result in a reduced oxygen supply to the cells.

Ginkgo is used to improve cerebrovascular insufficiency (reduced blood flow to the brain in the case of a stroke, ischaemic incidents and Alzheimer's disease), intermittent claudication (severe cramping in the legs during walking or exercise), tinnitus (ringing in the ears), vertigo (dizziness), impotence, Raynaud's disease and varicose ulcers.

Cerebrovascular insufficiency can lead to symptoms of depression, memory loss and confusion, which are often linked to cognitive degeneration in elderly people.

Results can be expected within eight to 12 weeks after commencing treatment with ginkgo.

Elderly people are very sensitive to prescription antidepressants and many people stop taking them because of the side effects. Research has shown that many depressive elderly people have a reduced blood flow to the brain. Ginkgo is very valuable in this respect, but the dosage should be increased to 120 mg twice a day. Improvement in state of mind, motivation and memory is sometimes observed after only four weeks of using ginkgo.

A dosage of 120 mg twice a day is recommended for Alzheimer's disease. Considerable research has shown that symptoms of Alzheimer's improve after only four weeks.

Ginkgo's side effect profile is very low. Fewer than 1 per cent of people get a mild upset stomach at first. People with cerebrovascular insufficiency sometimes get a slight headache which can last about 48 hours. This shows that the ginkgo is improving the flow of blood to the brain. Ginkgo shows no interaction with other medications; nor do the German Commission E monograph list any contraindications for the use of ginkgo during pregnancy and breastfeeding. German researchers compiled a series of monographs to document the research work they had done on herbal medicines and to set up specifications.

Hypericum (Hypericum perforatum, St John's wort, scull cap)
(About 700 mg a day in divided doses, i.e. 350 mg morning and evening; for major depression doses of up to 700 mg three times a day can be prescribed)

Hypericum (St John's wort, also known as curry bush and scull cap) has been used for decades for the treatment of infections, bruises, wounds, sunburn, ulcers, abscesses, leukaemia, arthritis, headaches, tension and digestive problems. Recent research, however, has highlighted hypericum as an extremely effective treatment of depression. Current research is investigating the use of hypericum for treating AIDS and cancer. It has potent antiviral properties and its photosensitive effect on certain people could be valuable in treating cancer. Photosensitivity makes cancer cells more sensitive to certain wavelengths of light so that radiation of cancer cells can be more effective. The hypericin in hypericum also suppresses the protein kinase enzymes that are responsible for cancer growth and the death of cells.

Hypericum contains more than ten other active ingredients that have pharmacological activity, including bioflavonoids and xanthones.

Hypericum is a garden plant in South Africa and is indigenous in parts of the Cape. In the United Kingdom it grows prolifically in the countryside. It can be taken as a tea by infusing five flowers in 250 m of boiling water.

Research has conclusively proven that hypericum is more effective than a placebo in treating mild depression and that it is at least as effective as the standard prescription antidepressants. The difference is that hypericum has fewer side effects than most antidepressants. Side effects can include digestive tract problems, allergic reactions, fatigue and photosensitivity (to sunlight). Conventional antidepressants include the above, as well as drowsiness, increase in (or loss of) body mass, headaches, epileptic seizures, loss of libido, dizziness, anxiety, difficulty in breathing, fever, palpitations and an underactive thyroid gland.

Hypericum probably carries out its antidepressant effect by increasing all the neurotransmitters that have to do with improved mood, namely dopamine, adrenalin, noradrenaline and serotonin. It acts as a selective reuptake inhibitor of all these substances. It should not be taken with other antidepressants as it could enhance the effects and side effects of prescription antidepressants. If you intend stopping your prescription antidepressants, do so under your doctor's supervision and do it gradually over a period of at least a month before you start using hypericum. The German Commission E monograph has set dosages of hypericum varying between 2 000 mg and 4 000 mg of the plant extract or 0,2-0,1 mg of hypericin a day. Usually 700-1 000 mg a day is sufficient to treat mild depression.

Beware of standard extracts that do not contain more than 0,3 percent hypericin. Researchers believed hypericin to be the most important ingredient in the treatment of depression. Current research has shown there are other, even more active, ingredients in curry bush (scull cap). However, should the concentration of hypericin get too high, too little of the other active ingredients will be present.

Kava *(Piper methysticum)*
(700-1 400 mg a day as required)

For centuries people on the islands of the Pacific Ocean (especially Fiji and the Polynesian Islands) have used kava or kava kava for its calming and stress-relieving properties. On a more spiritual level it improves the capacity for insight into the higher self and self-knowledge. In the Pacific Islands kava is known as the giver of peace and restfulness. Throughout the world there is great interest in the unique properties of kava. It has the ability to bring about a deep sensation of relaxation in the body, while allowing the mind to function more clearly (as happens in meditation).

The greatest advantage of kava is that it is has no documented side effects and it is not addictive. Long-term use can cause a yellowing of the skin, nails and hair. Allergic reactions are extremely rare.

Kava is used in the West as a sedative (especially in Europe where it is a registered medicine). Kava's effect can be favourably compared with that of the benzodiasepines (e.g. Valium, Xanor and Halcion), but without the side effects or danger of physical dependancy that these drugs have.

Kava also has pain-relieving and muscle-relaxant properties. It physically relieves the tension in muscles, but also works subtly on the subconscious to illuminate the cause of the tension so that it can be dealt with and processed.

Active ingredients in kava include the kava lactones kavain and dihydrokavain which have muscle relaxant, pain-relieving and sedative properties. Some of the other ingredients have antispasmodic properties (for cramps) and the yangonins are effective in treating disorders of the nervous system and to treat lack of concentration and failing memory. Make sure that the kava product you use is produced from extracts of the whole root. If only the top leaves of the plant are used, the psychological effect of kava is virtually absent.

Kava does not lead to feelings of euphoria (a high). It allows you to access certain parts of your mind, but you have to work at recognising the negative and suppressed emotions and experiences and work through them yourself. Kava should be taken over a period of time before you gradually become aware of its imperceptible, mind-enhancing properties.

Valerian root *(Valeriana officinalis)*
(About 300 mg capsules at night)

The German Commission E monograph describes valerian as a safe and effective sedative and tranquilliser for the treatment of anxiety, tension, restlessness and disturbed sleep. It can be used in the form of a tea, tincture, capsules or extract.

Valerian works in the same way as the benzodiasepines, but it does not cause listlessness, dullness, rebound depression or dependance. It is completely non-toxic, but it should not be used together with prescription sedatives or narcotics. There are no contraindications for taking valerian with alcohol or while driving or handling heavy machinery.

Remember that sleeping problems usually have a psychological origin. Herbs, B-complex vitamins and minerals such as calcium and magnesium may very well help you to sleep better, but they should be combined with stress management and relaxation techniques.

A good sleeping potion is a tea made of 10 g each of dried valerian root, lavender flowers, camomile flowers, lemon mint leaves *(Melissa officinalis)* and orange blossoms in boiling water with a bit of honey, taken just before bedtime. If you have these plants fresh in your garden, you can also use that for the tea. (Refer to page 159 for more details on the properties of medicinal herbs.)

13 Natural alternatives to antibiotics

The excessive use and abuse of antibiotics over the past few decades has led to great disillusionment and dissatisfaction. Throughout the world people began to realise that antibiotics were no longer the miracle cure for all infections. Bacteria became increasingly resistant to antibiotics. Various species also transferred this resistance to one another so that the resistance of one specific type of bacteria to an antibiotic could be transferred to bacteria of another species. This shows how well bacteria adapt to any threat to their species.

This resistance of bacteria to antibiotics should be seen as a favour to humankind rather than a tragedy. Researchers have been forced to call a halt to what now appears to be a move in the wrong direction and reconsider matters. This has helped us to take responsibility for our own health. We must educate ourselves and learn about the harmful side effects of all medication, not only antibiotics. As we become more aware that there are alternatives and excellent other options available to us, we can insist on using them as our first choice of treatment for all infections and other ailments and diseases. Antibiotics can be kept for the really serious bacterial infections; they will then be more effective and save lives. Research has shown that the resistance of bacteria to antibiotics will diminish very quickly as soon as antibiotics are used less frequently and more judiciously.

The problem of bacterial resistance is particularly serious in patients with a reduced immunity (for example after transplantation of kidneys and other organs, in AIDS patients and diabetics, during chemotherapy or after major surgery) where bacteria are resistant to even the most toxic antibiotics. Such patients are helpless in this situation and die as a result of overwhelming infection. Resistance is an enormous problem in hospitals today. Even tuberculosis is showing increasing resistance to medications that have previously been extremely effective.

It is no good saying that one individual who uses antibiotics as a preventive measure to guard against so called secondary infection is unlikely to lead to bacteria developing resistance. Anyone who uses antibiotics unnecessarily is adding to the problem of general resistance in the whole bacterial population. As responsible members of society, we all have a duty not to abuse antibiotics.

With the abuse of antibiotics every person's immune system shows an increasingly reduced resistance to bacterial and viral infections. Unless children are exposed to various foreign organisms, they will never develop a good general resistance to the different organisms and they will continually develop infections. These are prematurely treated unnecessarily with antibiotics and it becomes a vicious circle.

Antibiotics disturb the delicate balance between the essential bacteria and fungi in our digestive tract. Antibiotics destroy the normal flora in the intestines and the fungi gain dominance. This can lead to candida infections (thrush), a problem for many women as soon as they take antibiotics. Babies also get thrush if their bottles have been over sterilised. As soon as all the bacteria are destroyed, the fungi take over and thrush develops.

The normal population of bacteria in the digestive tract can be maintained by taking supplements of 'friendly' bacteria, called probiotics. If you suffer from any form of candida (vaginal, systemic or in the digestive canal) or have chronic diarrhoea, you can safely take *Lactobacillus acidophilus* or *Bifidobacterium bifidum* capsules to restore the balance in the digestive tract. These bacteria which occur naturally in the alimentary tract keep your immune system healthy; they produce vitamins (for example vitamin K) and help with the detoxification of environmental toxins and other substances. These functions are all very important for biochemical balance in the body. A diet of plenty of fruit and vegetables, wholegrain products, active-yeast dairy products (such as yoghurt) and a small amount of red meat promotes the growth of beneficial bacteria in the alimentary tract and protects the body from infections and carcinogens. Vitamins C and A, selenium and zinc also improve the body's natural resistance to infection. (Consult Chapter 5 on antioxidants.)

Another problem is that of allergic reactions to certain antibiotics, which occurs quite often and can vary from a light skin rash to an overwhelming shock reaction (anaphylaxis) which can be life-threatening.

Don't get me wrong! Modern technology and the development of antibiotics save lives every day. It is the injudicious use and abuse of antibiotics that cause problems. It is not sensible to treat every little infection with an antibiotic. In any event, antibiotics are ineffectual against viruses, fungi and parasites. About 90 per cent of all upper respiratory tract infections are caused by a virus. Only 2-5 per cent of these may develop into a secondary bacterial infection. Don't insist on an antibiotic because you have to attend an important meeting and want to prevent your infection from going any further. Rather use alternative remedies which are effective against bacteria, viruses, fungi and parasites - and support your immune system at the same time.

Many of the antibiotics we use today were developed from natural products in the first place. For example, Alexander Fleming accidentally discovered that the fungus penicillin kills bacteria. Since then modern technology has been able to isolate active ingredients from various plants, mass-produce them in a laboratory and take out patents to sell them at a great profit. Natural medicinal herbs are comparatively cheap; they cannot be patented and the profit margins involved are not as great. In isolating the active ingredients, the natural balance is disturbed. However, during the process of photosynthesis in the plant the energy of sunlight is converted into plant energy and by taking a whole-plant extract one takes in all the ingredients in perfect balance. If only active ingredients are isolated, the substances become too strong, the side effects increase dramatically and the natural plant energy is lost.

We are equipped with a very efficient immune system. If we give it opportunity and support, our immune system is quite capable of protecting us from nearly all outside invaders, including viruses and bacteria. We do not need antibiotics for every bacterial infection. Often an infection is simply the body's way of telling you that you are overdoing things – listen to your body. Take a few days off, relax, use supplements and natural, medicinal, well-researched herbal remedies and guide your body back to health.

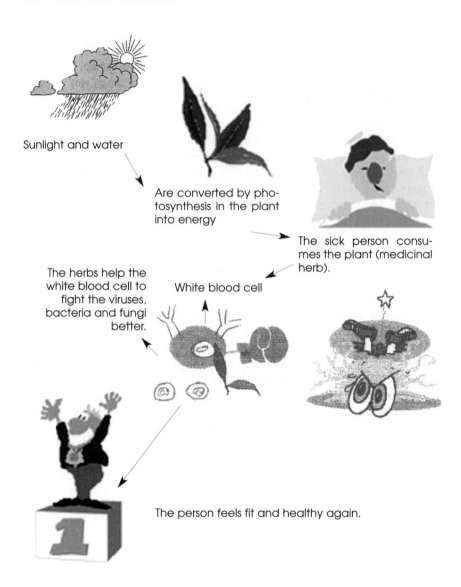

Sunlight and water

Are converted by photosynthesis in the plant into energy

The sick person consumes the plant (medicinal herb).

The herbs help the white blood cell to fight the viruses, bacteria and fungi better.

White blood cell

The person feels fit and healthy again.

Medicinal herbs

Let us discuss a few natural medicinal herbs. Thousands of plants are used as medicines. I have selected a few tried and tested examples which can help your body fight infection.

Remember that plants can also be harmful. Don't just use herbs from any source. If you have the knowledge, either make your own infusions from recognised herbs in your garden or use properly researched and well-known products from a reliable, established source. Consult one of the many health care providers who are knowledgeable in the use of medicinal herbs. Pregnant women and children should only take herbs recommended by trained experts. Most herbal plants are in fact quite safe – unlike many of the over-the-counter medicines and prescription drugs that we take in our ignorance without thinking any more about it. Always read the package inserts provided with conventional medication and find out about the possible side effects. Then make an informed decision on whether you want to use ordinary prescription medicines.

If you have an infection, use herbs until you feel better. The dosage and form (drops, tincture, dried leaves for a tea, etc.) will be indicated on the container or specifically prescribed. Stop taking the herbs as soon as you are well again. Many fresh herbs that we use with our food have medicinal value and, if used regularly, will be a good preventive measure against infection. Examples are rosemary, basil, thyme and garlic – to mention a few. Look out for products that contain combinations of herbs.

Standardised herb extracts are the best, followed by tinctures and then freeze-dried preparations. Herbal products are made from plants that have medicinal properties. Light, air and moisture affect dried plants and they lose their effectiveness. Plants react with oxygen and form free radicals; when plants are picked, they are no longer able to dispose of free radicals and the chemistry of the plant changes. Buy products that have been dried recently, preferably in light-resistant and airtight containers (dark-brown bottles or thick plastic containers). Before buying a herbal mixture, smell it. A strong smell indicates that the product is still fresh.

A standardised extract complies with the requirements for certain key ingredients in a product. Standardisation ensures that the product contains what it indicates and in sufficient quantities for the desired effect. It can be in liquid or solid form.

Tinctures are made by dissolving extracts of fresh or dried plants in alcohol. The alcohol content is high enough to preserve the plant matter. Remember that the quality of tincture is as good (or bad) as the herbs it contains. Shake tinctures well before using them and dissolve them in hot water. The usual dose is a dropper full in a quarter of a glass of water, taken three or four times a day with meals.

Freeze-drying is a process in which chemical solvents are used to make plant extracts. The extracts are then exposed to extremely low temperatures, thereby removing the solvents. The fixed residue is then packed in capsules. This process ensures products of a much better quality than whole air-dried plants.

It is not a good idea to use whole air-dried plants for medicinal purposes. If they are chopped fine and stored in a tin, they will probably lose all their healing powers. Leaves and flowers are especially prone to deterioration. If such herbs smell old, dusty or mouldy, they are probably of little value. Herbal teas must be very carefully packed to prevent deterioration and they should retain a strong, characteristic aroma. Try to buy organically grown herbal preparations. This ensures that poisons are eliminated and that natural compost has been used in their cultivation. Check the list of ingredients and make sure that no other pharmaceutical and potentially toxic substances have been added.

1 Echinacea, purple coneflower (*Echinacea purpurea* or *angustifolia* or *pallida*)

Echinacea is probably the most famous and best-researched immunostimulant herb in the world. It is widely used in preparations to treat the symptoms of colds and flu. It is also effective against any light to moderate infection.

Echinacea has been used by the North American Indians for centuries. Extensive clinical research is being conducted into its properties and thousands of doctors now use it to treat infections.

Its main applications include the following:

- Colds, flu, coughs, and other upper respiratory tract infections such as croup and bronchitis.
- Enlarged lymph glands, sore throat (streptococ bacteria) and tonsillitis.
- Toothache, mouth and gum infections – gargle with Echinacea and swallow it.

- Urinary tract infections: cystitis (infection of the bladder), urethritis (infection of the urethra) and prostatitis.
- Other mild infections and chronic infections such as chronic fatigue (yuppy flu or ME – myalgic encephalopathy). In Europe especially, Echinacea is used as a complementary therapy together with antibiotics and chemotherapy. It is particularly effective against infections where there is no chronic immune deficiency dysfunction.
- Herpes and candida infection – applied externally and taken per mouth.
- Applied externally to wounds, for skin infections (such as impetigo caused by staphylococcus), infections under the nails and for healing any persistent skin complaint or infection. Skin ulcers (such as varicose veins and diabetic ulcers) respond well if the affected area is kept covered with Echinacea. It is also effective for all insect bites and stings, even snakebite – applied externally and taken per mouth. Echinacea is excellent for boils, carbuncles, abscesses and acne – applied externally and taken per mouth.
- Blood and food poisoning – take high dosages every two hours.
- Burns – applied externally and taken per mouth.
- Pelvic infections.
- Psoriasis, eczema and inflammation of the skin – applied externally and taken per mouth.

General guidelines for dosage include the following:

- Use Echinacea three times a day while the infection persists.
- Echinacea root causes a slight numb sensation in the mouth. Put a drop of Echinacea on your tongue before you buy it. If it does not give you a numbing sensation on your tongue, it is not a good product. Try something else.
- The dried root can be used as a tea: 1-2 g three times a day.
- The freeze-dried plant can be used: 325-650 mg or three capsules three to four times a day.
- Echinacea tincture (1:5): 3-4 ml in water three times a day.
- Drops: 20-30 drops three times a day.
- Certain products contain Echinacea in combination with other antibacterial and anti-inflammatory herbs such as garlic, golden seal or hydrastis, yarrow, astragalus, sweet orange and camomile.

It is quite safe to use Echinacea. If you follow the dosages for adults and children (children under ten take half the recommended adult dose), there is no danger of toxicity. Echinacea can be used as a long-term supplement by people with a generally reduced immune activity - use half the dose for eight weeks and then leave it for a week. It is usually only necessary to use it for the duration of the disease.

Echinacea improves the non-specific activity of the immune system. It stimulates the general activity of white blood cells against any infective organisms. Unlike antibiotics, where bacteria are destroyed directly, Echinacea enables the immune cells to attack bacteria, viruses and other abnormal cells (such as cancer cells) more effectively and render them harmless.

More than 500 studies have been done documenting the chemical, pharmacological and clinical advantages of Echinacea. Echinacea stimulates phagocytosis in particular. This is the process whereby the scavenger white blood cells recognise foreign organisms, ingest them and then destroy them.

Echinacea's specific action in the body is described as follows:

- Echinacea increases the quantity and activity of all normal, mature white blood cells, including the antitumour cells.
- Echinacea promotes T-cell function. T-cells are white blood cells that are important for cell-mediated immunity. The T-cells are activated as soon as the B-cells (white blood cells with antibodies against specific foreign organisms or antigens on their cell membranes) link up with the foreign organism (or antigen). The T-cells then become killer cells that destroy the foreign organism. Cell-mediated immunity is particularly important for the body's resistance to bacteria, yeast cells and fungi such as Candida albicans, parasites and viruses (including Herpes simplex, Epstein-Barr and hepatitis). There are also T-helper cells which help the B-cells to make antibodies and T-suppressor cells which prevent the B-cells from making too many antibodies. Cell-mediated immunity is also responsible for protection against the development of cancer, autoimmune diseases (such as lupus and rheumatoid arthritis) and allergies. Echinacea is thus prescribed for all these conditions. In AIDS patients the T-cell function is suppressed. Ongoing research on the use of Echinacea as a treatment for AIDS is very promising.
- Echinacea stimulates the growth of new tissue to accelerate wound healing.
- Echinacea reduces inflammation in arthritis and skin disorders.
- Echinacea has mild antibiotic activity; it suppresses bacterial

growth; it is antiviral (suppresses viral growth) and antifungal (suppresses fungal growth).

- Echinacea suppresses the bacterial enzyme hyaluronidase which enables bacteria to destroy the cell membrane of healthy cells and enter the cell. This suppression of hyaluronidase probably accounts for Echinacea's efficacy against snakebite.

- Echinacea contains sterols and sterolins, the same active ingredients that are currently so popular in South Africa as a miracle cure for all ailments. These ingredients are only isolated from the African wild potato *(Hypoxis rooperi)* or pine nuts. (Pycnogenol is also made from pine bark or grape seed.) All plants contain sterols and sterolins, which are unfortunately destroyed in the cooking process. The sterols and sterolins are very potent immune system boosters. Like all medicinal plants (herbs), Echinacea also contains many other active ingredients (for example, polysaccharides, flavonoids such as quercetin, caffeic acid derivatives such as echinacosides, essential oils, polyacetylenes and alchylamines). That is why a whole-plant extract from a good, organically cultivated, reliable source is so much more beneficial than single, isolated active ingredients - as is the case with the new product that has been brought onto the market which contains only sterols and sterolins.

2 Garlic *(Allium sativum)*

Garlic is widely recognised as a culinary herb and a potent natural medicine that has improved people's health for centuries. Thousands of research studies done over the past 40 years have repeatedly proven the benefits of garlic. Garlic can be taken every day in the form of one or two cloves to treat high LDL-cholesterol, blood clots, hypertension and to prevent and treat all forms of infection. (Use fresh parsley as well to counter the strong odour!) If, however, you are already taking anticoagulants such as warfarin and aspirin, you should be careful not to eat too much garlic.

Fresh, finely chopped, is the best way to take garlic. The cooking process and the commercial production process of garlic destroy much of the natural activity that is present in the fresh plant. Fresh parsley disguises the odour problem associated with fresh garlic. Use finely chopped garlic in salads, salad dressings and other dishes. Capsules should be from a reliable source.

While garlic is a potent immune system booster, it is also an active antibiotic, an antifungal, antiparasitic, anti-inflammatory and a shield against radiation therapy. It has pain-relieving and antipyretic properties. Its active ingredients include alliin, which gives the garlic its characteristic taste and allicin, a sulphate which gives the garlic its characteristic odour. Garlic can be taken in large quantities to destroy foreign invaders such as viruses and bacteria without damaging the host in any way (the person who is eating the garlic!). During infection you can take a clove or capsule every three hours. Garlic is also effective against herpes infections (such as cold sores, genital herpes and chicken pox). All infections of the alimentary tract, including *Helicobacter pylori* which contributes to ulcers, respond well to garlic. Urinary tract and upper respiratory tract infections can also be well controlled with garlic. A little garlic oil on a piece of cottonwool can be used in an infected ear (for children and adults).

Make garlic oil by chopping garlic finely and soaking it for a few days in a little olive oil. Keep it in the fridge and warm up as needed. Garlic can also be added to food in this way. Some people put a whole clove of garlic in the ear canal, with a wad of cottonwool to keep it in position. It will eventually dissolve.

Garlic is also effective in treating Candida vaginalis and digestive tract infections (thrush). Garlic does not harm or destroy normal intestinal flora. It increases the secretion of bile and reduces spastic colon (it acts as an antispasmodic). Garlic is an effective expectorant; it loosens the mucous in the airways and promotes the expectoration of mucous in respiratory tract disorders.

3 Golden seal *(Hydrastis canadensis)*

Golden seal is probably the remedy of choice when it comes to anti-infective and anti-inflammatory herbs for the protection of all the mucous membranes in the body and hence for the treatment of disorders of the digestive tract, the eyes, airways, urinary tract and urogenital system. The North American Indians used this indigenous plant for hundreds of years before Western medicine discovered it.

One of the active ingredients in golden seal is berberine, which has antibacterial and immunostimulant properties. Golden seal is effective against a wide spectrum of bacteria and it contains antifungal activity as well. It will not cause an overgrowth of fungi, as happens with ordinary antibiotics.

Golden seal ensures the rapid recovery of the mucosal lining of the airways after infection. It reduces irritation of the mucosa of the digestive tract and is recommended for all disturbances of the alimentary tract such as poor digestion, gastritis, ulcers and infective diarrhoea.

At the first sign of a cold take golden seal as drops or as a tincture. It is successful in the treatment of haemorrhoids (piles), acne, eczema, bronchitis, bladder infections and candida, both as an external ointment and taken internally. It is a good antiseptic for dressing wounds. It can also be used as a gargle for sore throats and as a mouthwash for mouth ulcers, tonsillitis and gingivitis (gum infection). Golden seal is also a good vaginal douche for vaginal irritation. Dissolve golden seal in water as an effective eyewash for eye infections. Dissolve one capsule or quarter of a teaspoon of the powder in a cup of water. Strain it and use as described above.

Golden seal contains hydrastin which causes vascular constriction. People who are taking beta blockers such as Inderal should be careful with golden seal because it can complicate the regulation of blood pressure.

4 Astragalus *(Astragalus membranosus or Huang Qi)*

Astralagus is a well-known herb for the prevention of infections and to stop further deterioration in case of existing disease. It promotes the functioning of the body's immune system and forms the first line of defence between the body and the outside world. It protects us against bacteria and viruses and is best taken before infection has a chance to take hold. Use 20 drops twice a day for two or three months to support the immune system.

Astragalus is used particularly for the treatment of colds, flu and other respiratory tract infections. It is an adaptogen and supports the adrenal glands during times of stress. Long-term stress suppresses the immune system and infections are often the result.

5 Camomile *(Matricaria chamomilla)*

Camomile is valuable because it has three medicinal properties: it reduces inflammation, relieves muscle and abdominal spasm and reduces the abdominal swelling and pain associated with spasm. It is of particular value in treating bacterial gastroenteritis because of its ability to bind bacterial toxins and so perform an antibacterial action.

Camomile is generally used for the relief of cholic in babies and for stomach cramps. It is excellent for children and adults. It also has a calming effect.

Camomile can be taken as a tea or as drops for an upset stomach, poor digestion, tension and infections.

6 Thyme *(Thymus vulgaris)*

Thyme is used as a culinary herb but it is also an antiseptic, an antibacterial and antifungal agent. Its properties can be ascribed to its aromatic oils, thymol and carvacol. The volatile oils are excreted by the lungs so that thyme can be used effectively for all respiratory tract infections. Thyme is an excellent cough remedy, it helps to relax the bronchi (dilate them), it stimulates the immune system and fights viruses and bacteria. Thyme is also an excellent expectorant (it loosens the mucous and makes it easier to expectorate).

Thyme can be used as a gargle and mouthwash. However, it should not be used in large quantities by pregnant women as it could cause uterine contractions.

7 Elder flower *(Sambucus nigra)*

The flower of the elder tree is an antipyretic (it lowers fever by increasing the perspiration rate) and it is a general immunostimulant. The leaves can be applied externally to wounds and bruises, the bark is a diuretic (promoting the excretion of water by the kidneys) and the berries and flowers are used to treat colds and other respiratory tract infections by improving the body's resistance to infections.

8 Lime blossom *(Tilia cordata)*

In Europe especially, lime blossom is commonly used to treat colds, flu and coughs in children. It contains many plant chemicals which reduce the congestion of the bronchial tree.

Lime blossom is also an immunostimulant. In a study comparing the effect of lime blossom to an ordinary antibiotic in treating respiratory tract infections, lime blossom tea was found to be much more effective than antibiotics in reducing the duration and severity of infections.

9 Cranberry *(Vaccinium macrocarpon)*

The juice of the cranberry is very effective in the treatment and pre-vention of all urinary tract infections. Recent studies have shown that this is a safe, effective treatment for dealing with bladder, urethra and kidney infections in the short and long term. Cranberry juice reduces the ability of bacteria to attach to the bladder wall, thereby inhibiting bacterial growth.

10 Ginger *(Gingiber officinalis)*

Ginger has anti-inflammatory, painkilling, antipyretic and antibacteri-al properties. It slows down the body's production of pain-generating chemicals such as leukotrines and certain prostaglandins.

11 Sage *(Salvia officinalis)*

The use of sage as a medicinal herb dates from the time of the Ancient Greeks. Sage contains tannins (as found in red wine) which reduce the inflammation associated with sore throats. It also has strong antibacte-rial properties and is a good gargle and mouthwash for treating throat infections.

12 Liquorice root *(Glycyrrhiza alba)*

Liquorice root has been used for more than 3 000 years to treat many ailments. It is often used for respiratory tract infections and sore throats because of its pain-relieving effects and its antibacterial and antiviral properties. Liquorice root is also an anti-inflammatory and acts as an antioxidant. Studies show that it also protects the liver against the hepatitis-C virus infection that sometimes lead to cancer of the liver.

Liquorice root contains glycericine which can stimulate steroid activ-ity when taken in very large quantities. This may lead to metabolic dis-turbances (potassium loss, oedema, hypertension and increased body mass)

However, it can be safely used for four to six weeks in moderate amounts in the forms of a tea, tincture or drops for treating upper respiratory tract infections. Liquorice root is also an adaptogen.

13 Buchu *(Agathosma betulina)*

Buchu tea, made from an indigenous South African plant, is effective in treating kidney stones, bladder infection, blood in the urine, any chronic urinary tract disorders and arthritis. Buchu also has moderate antidiuretic and antiseptic properties. It is very safe to use. All urinary tract complaints should be discussed with a medical doctor, especially if there is blood in the urine.

14 Other herbs

Yarrow, aloe (aloe vera), milk thistle (contains silymarine), peppermint, cayenne pepper (red chilli pepper containing capsaicin which activates the pain nerves and then has the effect of a local anaesthetic), turmeric (contains curcumin), lemon peel, lemon verbena and orange peel all have anti-inflammatory properties which help alleviate the muscle pains and fever associated with infections and inflammation. Most of these have antioxidant properties which boost the immune system and improve general resistance to infections.

The active ingredients in medicinal herbs have the ability to penetrate into the inner core of every cell and repair functions deep within the cell and the subcellular structures in a very subtle way. Herbs even act on the transfer of messages in the nervous system and affect the way we feel, the way every system in the body works and the way we think. Scientists are only now starting to discover by means of nanotechnology and quantum physics just how subtle the effects of medicinal herbs really are. They are a wonderful gift from our Creator and we should use them with reverence, responsibility, respect and compassion for the wellbeing of our mind and body.

USE MEDICINAL HERBS CAREFULLY AND WITH
THE NECESSARY KNOWLEDGE. IT IS IMPORTANT
TO REALISE WHEN A HERB IS NOT WORKING AND
THEN TO SEEK ADDITIONAL THERAPY. HOWEVER,
HERBS ARE ONE OF THE BEST WAYS TO HANDLE
MOST COMMON INFECTIONS. MEDICINAL HERBS
ARE USUALLY SAFE, EFFECTIVE AND EASY TO USE,
WITH FEW SIDE EFFECTS.

Case study

Pierre was five when his mother brought him for a consultation. He
was a premature baby and kept getting respiratory tract infections. As
a baby he spent more time in hospital than at home and even as a toddler at least once a month he had to spend a night in the casualty ward
or be admitted to the paediatric ward for a few days with croup, asthma or pneumonia. He was a miserable, sickly child who could not participate in sport. His appetite was poor and he was small for his age. He
had eczema, sporadic bouts of candida infection in the mouth (thrush),
coupled with diarrhoea and he showed intolerance to various types of
food. Winters were a nightmare. His parents were desperate. He would
have to go to school soon and they had no idea how he would ever
cope.

Pierre's medication for the six months prior to this consultation
(only two of which were winter months) was as follows:

22/01: Cephalosporin (antibiotics)
Cortisone-antihistamine combination
Anti-inflammatory, antipyretic medication with paracetamol,
codeine and ibuprofen

14/02: Amoxyllin and clavulinic acid (antibiotics)
Antihistamine and painkiller

15/03: Erythromycin (antibiotics)
Cortisone-antihistamine combination
Anti-inflammatory, antipyretic medication

30/03: Trimethoprim and sulphamethoxazole (antibiotics)
Cough mixture with expectorant and bronchodilator

10/04: Cephalosporin (antibiotics)
Cough mixture with codeine and antihistamine
Pain syrup with codeine and paracetamol

08/05: Amoxycillin and clavulinic acid (antibiotics)

16/05: Amoxycillin and clavulinic acid (antibiotics)
Cortisone-antihistamine combination

10/06: Cephalosporin (antibiotics)
Pain syrup

28/06: Erythromycin (antibiotics)
Cortisone-antihistamine combination

With all this medication it was not surprising that the child had no re-sistance. Continuous use of antibiotics may lead to eczema, allergies and food intolerance. The diarrhoea and lack of appetite were caused by antibiotic abuse, with consequent overproduction of intestinal can-dida causing an infected mucosa, poor absorption and a chronic feel-ing of fatigue and malaise. The excessive use of cortisone resulted in metabolic disturbances, fatigue and a water and electrolyte imbalance. The antihistamines made him feel tired and over dried the mucosa, resulting in the production of more mucous to cope with the irritation. This in turn made the upper respiratory tract infection worse.

All prescription medication was stopped. I prescribed a good gener-al vitamin and mineral supplement to boost the immune system (con-taining mainly antioxidants with iron, chromium, B-complex vitamins, copper, zinc and vanadium). Pierre also took essential fatty acids (gamma linolenic and eicosapentaenoic acids) with calcium and mag-nesium. These combinations became his daily supplements. (Consult Chapter 14 on the respiratory system.)

To support his immune system and get rid of the viruses, bacteria and fungi, inflammation and thick mucous, he took a combination of Echinacea, garlic, golden seal, astragalus, yarrow, bromelain (pineapple extract), lime blossom and camomile four times a day for two weeks and then twice a day for four weeks. For three days his mother made him a warm drink at night with lukewarm water, one tablespoon of honey, a pinch of turmeric and ginger, with freshly chopped sage and thyme in it to loosen the mucous and relieve the sore throat. Pierre also took *Lactobacillus acidophilus* powder to restore the balance in the digestive tract so that the normal intestinal flora (bacteria) could be restored and to prevent the candida and fungi from overgrowing.

While his appetite was poor, he took an amino acid powder with the necessary carbohydrates, micronutrients and fats as a food substitute.

Within two weeks Pierre was a different child. He developed an enormous appetite and ran around happily. Every night in his prayers he thanked Jesus for his exciting new life. Pierre is now in Grade 2. He is doing well at school and participates in every sport. During the past two years he only needed antibiotics once – for a bad bout of bronchitis. As soon as he shows signs of a cold, his mother increases his antioxidant supplements. She always keeps a supply of the herbal combination so that she can give it to him for a few days when necessary.

14 Micronutrients for the respiratory system

Probably the most common reason for consulting a doctor or any other health care professional is disorders of the respiratory system. Most people suffer from colds, flu, sinusitis, bronchitis or pneumonia at least once a year, usually in winter. Allergies of the respiratory tract (such as hay fever and sinusitis) are the most common form of allergy among children and adults. Chronic postnasal drip, ear infections and tonsillitis are common causes of illness among young children and adults. Chronic bronchitis and emphysema affect many older people.

If you take antibiotics for every respiratory tract infection or problem, you will soon end up in a vicious circle of lowered resistance and re-infection. The usual prescription medication for asthma, chronic bronchitis and emphysema have many side effects and seldom cure the condition. Upper respiratory tract infections are often a sign that you're overdoing things. Don't insist on antibiotics and antihistamines. Rather take a few days' leave and give your body a chance to recover. Drink plenty of fluids, drink fresh fruit and vegetable juice, dissolve eucalyptus oil in boiling water and steam those sinuses, take 2 000 mg of vitamin C and herbs (as described in Chapter 13) and you will soon recover. A good gargle for sore throats is sage tea.

Try this recipe for colds, thick mucous and sinusitis: Mix a pinch of ginger, cinnamon, mustard, cayenne pepper and turmeric with a fresh clove of garlic (optional), a little lemon juice and honey in lukewarm water. Add a pinch of sage and thyme if the mucous is yellow or green. Drink this regularly until you feel better. The same applies to people with chronic lung problems. A good micronutrient supplement, with the correct stress management, will certainly improve the condition, or at least alleviate it and reduce the duration and frequency of acute outbreaks.

If you start taking supplements, don't just throw out all your prescription medications. Keep taking them. You and your doctor will soon discover that you can reduce the dosage or change to a milder product. Asthma sufferers will find that they use their inhalers much less and have fewer episodes of acute bronchospasm. Children will have fewer middle-ear infections, bouts of tonsillitis and colds. Be patient, use your supplements every day and you will get better.

Keep the antibiotics for serious, persistent and life-threatening infections and they will be much more effective. Remember that up to 95 per cent of upper respiratory tract infections are caused by a virus and only 2-5 per cent develop into secondary bacterial infections. Don't take antibiotics too soon. Even the most severe bacterial infections can be cured without antibiotics by using an immune-boosting supplement and medicinal herbs.

Micronutrients for optimal wellbeing of the respiratory system

1 Vitamins and minerals
(Children under ten use half the adult dosage)

- Vitamin A (15 000 IU or 4 545 micrograms or 4,5 mg of RE a day during the acute phase; then reduce to 5 000 IU or 1 515 micrograms of RE a day for maintenance). Vitamin A protects the mucous lining in the respiratory system and ensures its rapid recovery after infections. It also improves immunity by stimulating the antibody reaction and supporting the function of white blood cells. In supporting the mucosa, vitamin A also protects the respiratory tract against the irritating effects of smoke and other pollutants in the airways. Vitamin A forms the first line of defence against the invasion of harmful bacteria, viruses and fungi.
- Beta carotene and other carotenoids (25 000 IU or 15 mg a day during the acute phase; then reduce to the maintenance dose of 15 000 IU or 10 mg a day). Beta carotene is converted into vitamin A as and when the body needs it, but has antioxidant properties of its own. Beta carotene protects the respiratory system against the damage by free radicals caused by smoke, pollution, inhaled toxins and allergens (substances that induce an allergic reaction in sensitive people).
- Vitamin D (400 IU a day). Together with vitamin A, vitamin D reduces the frequency of asthma attacks and the duration of a respiratory tract infection. Vitamin D plays an important role in the treatment and prevention of allergies. (Consult Chapter 10 on calcium, magnesium and vitamin D.)

- Vitamin E and selenium (200 IU or 166 mg of vitamin E and 100 micrograms of selenium a day). As an antioxidant, vitamin E is important in supporting the immune system and destroying free radicals. Vitamin E is also involved in the control of allergies by enabling the immune system to react more normally thereby reducing the abnormal reaction to innocent invaders (such as house mite and pollen), a typical characteristic of allergies. (Consult Chapter 5 on antioxidants.)

  Vitamin E supports lung function by improving oxygen supply to the lungs. It protects the mucous membranes and accelerates recovery after·the mucosa has been damaged during infection, exposure to smoke and allergies of the respiratory tract.

  Vitamin E improves the immunity to viruses and bacteria. It is especially important against herpes infections such as shingles, chicken pox, cold sores and genital herpes.

- Vitamin C (2 000 mg a day in four divided doses during the acute phase; then reduced to 250-500 mg a day morning and evening for maintenance). This vitamin is probably best-known for treating colds and flu. During the 1960s Linus Pauling proved that vitamin C reduces the duration, frequency and severity of upper respiratory tract infections, cancer and allergies.

  Vitamin C supports the immune system in cases of chronic respiratory tract infection and helps the body to fight against viruses, bacteria and fungi.

  Vitamin C is a natural antihistamine that prevents and reduces the overproduction of histamine by the mast cells (white blood cells that are intimately involved in allergic reactions). It is extremely important in all allergies of the respiratory system – and there are no side effects such as drowsiness or dehydration of the mucosa, which are often typical of the prescription antihistamines.

  Vitamin C also has an anti-inflammatory effect that reduces the inflammation process in the respiratory tract.

- B-complex vitamins (about 50 mg of each and 50 micrograms of B12) including thiamine, riboflavin, pantothenic acid, pyridoxine and cobalamin. Thiamine (B1) can contribute to breaking a fever and is also valuable for treating respiratory tract infections. Riboflavin (B2) improves and supports the oxygen supply to cells and is useful for treating allergies of the respiratory tract. Pantothenic acid (B5) helps to alleviate allergies of the respiratory tract, asthma and infections through the support given to the respiratory system by co-enzyme A. Pyridoxine (B6) helps in coping with and treating

asthma, allergies and infections. Cobalamin (B12) improves children's appetites and helps for allergies, asthma and viral infections.
- Calcium (about 100 mg in amino acid chelation or food form for the respiratory system; more for the prevention of osteoporosis) improves and alleviates all allergic symptoms. (Consult Chapter 10 on the role of calcium.) Where allergies are a factor (as in asthma and hay fever), it reduces the duration and frequency of respiratory problems.
- Magnesium (about 50 mg in chelation or food form for the respiratory system) alleviates bronchospasm (contraction of the bronchial tubes) by relaxing the smooth muscle of the bronchi.
- Zinc (15 mg in chelation form) improves the general immunity to viral and bacterial infections. It reduces the duration and frequency of respiratory tract infections. Zinc (gluconate) lozenges are excellent for a sore throat. Zinc is generally used in the treatment of colds and flu.

2 Amino acids

- Histidine (100 mg a day) stimulates tissue repair after injury (for example after infections, allergies and damage from smoking). Histidine reduces and controls the production of histamine, an important function for treating allergies and infections.
- Tyrosine (100 mg a day) has a moderate antioxidant effect and neutralises free radicals caused by smoking and stress. Stress exacerbates allergies (especially asthma and eczema) and in many cases even causes the allergy. Tyrosine is an important precursor in the production of the stress hormones (cortisol and adrenalin). Tyrosine improves the body's capacity to handle and cope with stress and is often used to treat stress-related anxiety attacks. It reduces the physical and psychological impact of stress and hence the allergic reaction and the chance of infections.
- N-acetyl-L-cysteine (NAC, 250 mg a day), an amino acid that contains sulphates, is involved in the synthesis of glutathione, a strong antioxidant and detoxifying substance. (Consult Chapter 5 on antioxidants.) It protects the lungs against damage from free radicals caused by smoke and pollution.

  NAC also breaks down the bonds that are responsible for the thickening of mucous during allergies and infection and makes the mucous easier to expectorate. It is especially important for the long-term treatment of lung problems such as asthma, chronic bronchitis and emphysema. NAC can also be used in higher doses of 500-1 000 mg a day by children affected by cystic fibrosis.

NAC also has an antiviral effect. It increases the levels of glutathione in virus-infected cells thereby preventing the spread of viruses.

NAC is commonly used for the treatment of all disorders of the respiratory system, smoker's cough, asthma, psoriasis and cancer. Together with beta carotene, selenium and zinc, it protects the alveoli (tiny air sacs where exchange of oxygen and carbon dioxide takes place) from smoke damage.

3 Essential fatty acids

The omega-3 and omega-6 fatty acids are effective supplements for all respiratory tract infections and allergies. They improve immunity and are recommended for chronic respiratory problems such as asthma, chronic bronchitis, sinusitis, cystic fibrosis and allergies. (Consult Chapter 9 on essential fatty acids for more information on dosages, etc.)

4 Medicinal herbs for the respiratory tract

The most important herbs for all disorders of the airways are Echinacea, garlic, astragalus, golden seal, lime blossom, sage, elder flower, thyme and liquorice root. (Consult Chapter 13 on natural alternative to antibiotics.) Most of these herbs help to reduce mucous, help the mucosal lining to recover more quickly after infection and are also effective against viruses, bacteria, fungi and parasites. Most of them also strengthen the immune system. Garlic has a high NAC content that makes it very effective in reducing mucous in colds and flu. Mustard also contains a lot of NAC. Turmeric contains curcumin which has a strong antiviral and anti-inflammatory effect.

- Wild cherry bark is often used to treat an irritating, consistent cough that keeps you awake at night. It is also good for people who suffer from chronic bronchitis and for whooping cough. One of its ingredients is prunacin, a light cough suppressant and antispasmodic. Take 20-30 drops of the extract or one teaspoon of the cough mixture every three hours.

- Pineapple extract (containing the enzyme bromelain) is a potent anti-inflammatory with mucolytic (to break down mucous) and antibacterial properties. It also improves the efficacy of prescription antibiotics and reduces the infection of the sinuses and bronchial tubes.
- Quercetin, one of the bioflavonoids, accelerates the recovery of the mucosa after infection. It also has an anti-inflammatory and antiviral effect. Quercetin stabilises the granulation of the mast cells and basophils (the white blood cells involved in allergic reactions) and prevents the release of histamine. In this respect it acts as a natural antihistamine (like vitamin C) and reduces the duration and frequency of allergic reactions.
- Feverfew *(Chrysanthemum parthenium)* has been used for thousands of years as a fever-reducing substance and painkiller. It also helps for migraine and muscle spasm. People who are taking anticoagulants such as warfarin and aspirin should be careful when using feverfew and come off it gradually to avoid rebound blood clotting.

These are a few of the best-known herbs on which considerable research has been done. There are many other Chinese, African, American and European herbs that are commonly used to treat respiratory problems.

These guidelines should not be seen as an attempt to replace medical advice. If natural remedies and supplements do not improve the condition within three days, or if the condition gets worse, consult your doctor at once. An acute asthma attack, croup, and pneumonia (infection of the lungs) are examples of diseases where Western medicine and today's technology can be utilised to best advantage and save lives.

Case studies

Two brothers, Johan (now aged eight) and Etienne (now six), have had respiratory problems since birth. Johan gets asthma and Etienne regularly gets middle-ear infection (otitis media) and tonsillitis. Their medical history (consultation with doctors and medication) is a real horror story.

Name	Consultation	Diagnosis	Medication
Etienne 12/03/95	Paediatrician	Tonsillitis	Antibiotics Decongestant Painkiller
Etienne 16/03/95	Paediatrician	Bronchitis	Antibiotics Decongestant mixture Cortisone-antihistamine combination
Etienne 05/05/95	General practitioner	Acute middle-ear infection	Antibiotics Painkiller Cortisone-antihistamine combination
Etienne 26/07/95	General practitioner	Tonsillitis	Antibiotics Decongestant mixture Painkiller
Johan 28/07/95	Paediatrician	Asthma	Nebuliser Inhalation Cortisone Antibiotics X-rays (chest)
Johan 30/07/95	Casualty	Paediatrician	Acute bronchospasm Nebuliser Inhalation Bronchodilator (injection) Cortisone
Etienne 08/08/95	General practitioner	Middle-ear infection	Antibiotics
Etienne 09/08/95	Paediatrician	Middle-ear infection	Broad-spectrum antibiotics Cortisone-antihistamine combination
Johan 15/08/95	Hospital	Acute broncho-spasm	Nebuliser Cortisone Antibiotics

Name	Consultation	Diagnosis	Medication
Etienne 19/09/95	Hospital	Grommets in ears	Antibiotics
Johan 19/09/95	General practitioner	Bronchospasm	Nebuliser
Etienne 13/10/95	Pharmacy	Common cold	Decongestant mixture
Etienne 20/10/95	Paediatrician	Middle-ear infection	Antibiotics Decongestant mixture Painkiller
Etienne 05/11/95	General practitioner	Tonsillitis	Antibiotics Decongestant mixture Painkiller
Johan 10/11/95	Paediatrician	Asthma	New nebuliser - use three times a day
Johan 25/11/95	General practitioner	Bronchitis	Antibiotics Cortisone-antihistamine combination
Etienne 27/11/95	Ear, nose and throat specialist	Middle-ear infection	Antibiotics

In February 1996 both boys were put onto a natural alternative to antibiotics for three weeks, together with a supplement to boost the respiratory system and additional calcium, magnesium, vitamin C and essential fatty acids, which they had to take every day.

Name	Consultation	Diagnosis	Medication
Johan 01/06/96	General	Common cold	Double dose of supplements for respiratory problems and natural alternatives to antibiotics
Etienne 05/07/96	ENT specialist	Middle-ear infection	Antibiotics
Johan 22/07/96	Paediatrician	Bronchitis	Antibiotics
Etienne 01/08/96	ENT specialist	Tonsillitis	Antibiotics
Etienne 23/10/96	Paediatrician	Mild asthma attack	Bronchodilator – inhaler
Johan 21/11/96	Pharmacy	Common cold mild asthma	Antibiotics Painkiller and anti-inflammatory
Etienne 20/01/97	ENT specialist	Middle-ear infection	Double dose of supplements for respiratory problems and natural alternatives to antibiotics

Etienne 23/02/97	Paediatrician	Middle-ear infection	Antibiotics Cortisone-antihistamine combination
Etienne 10/04/97	Hospital	Tonsillectomy	
Etienne 24/04/97	Paediatrician	Middle-ear infection	Antibiotics
Johan 29/08/97	General practitioner	Common cold, mild asthma	Decongestant mixture
Etienne 15/10/97	ENT specialist	Middle-ear infection	Antibiotics

As soon as a cycle of antibiotics is started, the immune system is suppressed and more infections follow. The vicious circle has to stop somewhere! After another consultation I persuaded the boys' mother to stop the medication and all doctors' consultations for two months and let the children take only the respiratory supplements, natural antibiotics, calcium supplement and essential fatty acids. Johan was to use his inhaler only if his chest closed up (in other words, on demand). From that time to the time of writing their only medical consultations have been to the dentist, occupational therapist (Johan had slight attention deficit which improved remarkably with the correct supplementation) and speech therapist (because of his middle-ear infection Etienne developed a speech problem because the infections affected his hearing).

Johan's acute asthma attacks decreased dramatically after February 1996 and from June 1997 to June 1999 he used only two cartridges of his nebuliser and one cartridge of his cortisone inhaler. Etienne's infections also began to improve after November 1995 and have now virtually stopped. If the children get sick, their supplements are doubled and they use natural alternatives to antibiotics for a week or two. The family's health insurance claims have also decreased dramatically and all their medical expenses are much less. The cost of the supplements is about a tenth of the other medication and there are no side effects. In fact, besides supporting the respiratory system and preventing infection, the supplements have had a positive effect on the whole body and general state of mind. Both children look well and feel great. This cannot only be ascribed to the fact that most children outgrow their respiratory problems as they grow older.

15 Special needs for special situations

15.1 Pregnancy and breastfeeding

These two subjects are inseparable and are therefore discussed together. The mother's micronutrient status is important even before she falls pregnant. Throughout the pregnancy the micronutrient status should remain optimal for the health of the growing foetus and for the mother's own wellbeing. Micronutrients remain important to both mother and child throughout the breastfeeding period, and then on through the toddler stage, the childhood and teenage years. (Consult 15.2 for the special needs of children and teenagers.)

Good nutrition before and during pregnancy can make a great difference to your baby's health and general wellbeing for the rest of its life. Eat healthy nutritious food, concentrating on fruit and vegetables, wholegrain products (the fibre is needed to prevent constipation during pregnancy), fish and chicken. The pregnant woman's body needs more of everything: proteins, carbohydrates, mono- and polyunsaturated fats (you need about 10 500 kilojoules or 2 500 calories a day), calcium, iron, zinc, all the B-complex vitamins, antioxidants and most of the other vitamins and minerals. An average increase of 12 kg in body mass ensures a healthy mother and baby.

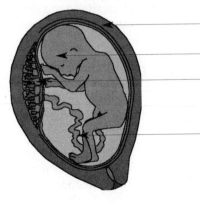

Uterus (womb)

Foetus (developing embryo)

Placenta of uterus through which the nutrients and oxygen are passed from mother to foetus.

Umbilical cord carrying all the nutrients, including micronutrients
and oxygen to the foetus and taking back all the waste products and carbon
dioxide back to the placenta for excretion.

During pregnancy and breastfeeding there is a good chance of developing marginal vitamin and mineral deficiencies. If a woman tends towards a marginal deficiency before pregnancy, the greater demands of pregnancy may result in a deteriorating marginal deficiency or even a fullblown vitamin deficiency in both mother and baby. Six months before you plan to fall pregnant, check that your health is in peak condition. The same applies to your husband (for healthy, good quality sperm). Make sure that you are not anaemic and see that your lifestyle is healthy. Exercise regularly, take your daily supplements, drink at least eight glasses of water a day, don't smoke, use alcohol moderately or not at all and practise relaxation techniques. Meditation and yoga are ideal activities to ensure a serene and joyful pregnancy. These are simply good habits that will enable you and your family to enjoy a lifetime of good health and wellbeing. A healthy diet with good supplementation will also prevent most of the pregnancy cravings for something sweet, sour or bitter – which is usually the body's way of finding a specific micronutrient.

Micronutrients and marginal deficiencies

- Folic acid supplements before and during pregnancy have numerous benefits. They are essential for the development of the nervous system and they prevent neural tube defects. What is less widely known is the fact that mothers with children who have neural tube disorders have a weakened function of the enzyme methionine synthetase. This causes an accumulation of homocysteine which can lead to nerve damage in the developing foetus. (Read the section on homocysteine in Chapter 5 on antioxidants.) In addition to folic acid, vitamins E, B6 and B12 are also essential to the functioning of this enzyme. It is therefore essential to take folic acid (800 micrograms), vitamin E (200 IU), vitamin B6 (50 mg) and B12 (100 micrograms) in your supplement before and during pregnancy. Use it while you are breastfeeding too. Folic acid is also important for the formation of red blood cells in the foetus, as well as the growth and division of other body cells.
- Calcium is essential for the growing foetus. Unless you take extra calcium during pregnancy, it is removed from your bones for the foetus' needs. The foetus needs calcium for the development of bones and teeth, muscles and heart, normal blood clotting and neuron transfer. Eat foods rich in calcium such as fish, dairy products,

wholegrain, nuts, seeds, green leafy vegetables and other vegetables. Supplement this with 600 mg of calcium in an amino acid chelation or food form or as a lactate or gluconate and take 300 mg of magnesium as well. If your intake of dairy products is low or nil, take at least 900 mg of calcium and 450 mg of magnesium a day. This will prevent painful Braxton-Hicks contractions as well as muscular pains and spasms. Remember to take your calcium and magnesium at night for a better night's rest. This works very well late in the pregnancy. Keep up the supplementation while you are breastfeeding and afterwards to prevent osteoporosis.

A craving for salt or pickled things to nibble is often caused by a lack of sodium. Eat foods that are rich in sodium such as celery, beetroot, cheese and eggs. Use vegetable salt or sea salt moderately. Cravings for non-specific things usually indicate a need for more water.

- Iron is an important micronutrient during pregnancy and breastfeeding. A woman's need for iron increases dramatically when she is pregnant. Iron is essential for the formation of red blood cells in both the mother and the foetus, and it prevents anaemia. It also helps to prevent disease and increase resistance. Take supplemental of about 30 mg of iron a day. Iron is poorly absorbed and it is usually necessary to take more (about 60 mg). This sometimes causes nausea and black stools, during pregnancy – the last thing a pregnant woman feels like coping with! However, if you take iron in an amino acid chelation or food form, 30 mg a day will be quite sufficient because the iron is absorbed so much better. The lower dose will also prevent the nausea and black stools. Good sources of iron include liver, red meat, eggs, chicken, salmon, kelp (marine algae), brewer's yeast, molasses, prunes, peanuts, mushrooms, spinach, nuts, seeds and pulses.

- Zinc is also important for the normal development of the immune system. Take a zinc supplement in an amino acid chelation or food form: 20 mg a day during pregnancy and breastfeeding. A marginal deficiency, especially in premature babies, can often cause nappy rash and diarrhoea. A zinc supplement will improve this dramatically.

You can also take an antioxidant vitamin and mineral supplement to balance the increased metabolism (more free radicals) during pregnancy and to support the immune system of both mother and baby.

Guidelines for using supplements during pregnancy and breastfeeding

1 Multivitamin and antioxidant combination

Antioxidants will accelerate wound healing after a Caesarian section or the episiotomy incision after a normal delivery and reduce the chances of scarring and secondary infection. Use a tissue oil that contains vitamins A, C and E with wheatgerm, avocado, jojoba and almond oil before and after the Caesarian section. Mix tissue oil with aloe vera, calendula and camomile to prevent or reduce stretch marks. (Consult Chapter 5 on supplements and antioxidants.)

Don't worry if the combination you choose has a little less of some of the ingredients. What is important is to see that you are taking most of these ingredients – as long as the quantities are not a lot less than the recommended intake.

- Vitamin A, 8 000 IU (2 424 RE) a day
- Beta carotene and other carotenes, 15 000 IU (10 mg) a day
- Vitamin C, 1 000 mg a day (in divided doses; the evening dose together with a calcium and magnesium supplement)
- Vitamin E, 200 IU (166 mg) a day
- Selenium, 100 micrograms a day
- Vitamins B1, B2, B3, B5, B6, 50 mg of each a day
- Vitamin B12, 100 micrograms a day
- Folic acid, 800 micrograms a day
- Biotin, 200 micrograms a day
- Choline, 50 mg a day
- Inositol, 50 mg a day
- Bioflavonoids, 100 mg a day
- Chromium, 200 micrograms a day
- Copper, 2 mg a day
- Iodine, 100 micrograms a day
- Iron, 30 mg a day
- Manganese, 2 mg a day
- Molybdenum, 30 micrograms a day
- Potassium, 100 mg a day
- Zinc, 20 mg a day

2 Calcium and magnesium supplements

The following quantities are recommended:

- Calcium, 600-900 mg a day
- Magnesium, 300-450 mg a day
- Vitamin D, 400 IU a day – especially important during breastfeeding
- Vitamin C, 200 mg a day

(Consult Chapter 10 on the role of calcium and magnesium.)

3 Essential fatty acids

The omega-3 fatty acid docosahexanoic acid (DHA) is particularly important for the development of the unborn foetus, baby and young child. DHA is essential for the development of the brain and the visual reaction of the eyes to light. It occurs in high concentrations in the photoreceptors of the retina and provides the retinal membranes with lipids. This ensures that the baby can clearly distinguish fine differences between light and dark. This in turn means that babies are soon able to interpret facial expressions and features. The foetus gets DHA and other essential fatty acids from the mother. After birth the baby takes these supplements in through the breast milk or a milk formula. The mother's intake thus determines whether the baby will have sufficient essential fatty acids.

The most important aspect of brain development occurs during the first few weeks of embryonic development, often before the woman even knows she is pregnant. After the second month the brain grows at an amazing rate and even after birth 60 per cent of the baby's energy is allocated to nourishing the brain. Supplements of essential fatty acids are a must for the mother and the baby who is using a milk formula that does not contain any essential fatty acids.

The best dietary sources of the omega-3 fatty acids are salmon, mackerel, tuna, sardines, trout, flax oil, pumpkin seeds, soya beans (plant oils also contain omega-6 fatty acids) and the dark-green vegetables (also a source of omega-6 fatty acids). Soya milk is therefore a good source of essential fatty acids for babies.

Much research is currently being conducted on the correct quantities of alpha linolenic acid, docosahexanoic acid and eicosapentanoic acid to add to milk formula and the correct ratio between omega-6 and omega-3 fatty acids. This ratio ensures that the balance between the formation of arachidonic acid and docosahexanoic acid is correct.

A general guideline to supplementation during pregnancy and breastfeeding is:

- Gamma linolenic acid (omega-6), 250 mg a day (about 1 000 mg of evening primrose oil)
- Eicosapentaenoic acid and docosahexanoic (omega-3), together about 300 mg a day of salmon oil.

These amounts are also suitable for babies, children and teenagers. (Consult Chapter 9 on essential fatty acids.)

15.2 Children and teenagers

Considerable research indicates that supplementary micronutrients improve the function of the nervous system, the immune system and the endocrine system in growing children, resulting in better cognitive functions (memory, concentration, eye-hand co-ordination and non-verbal intelligence). Non-verbal intelligence is considered an indication of basic physiological functioning in which micronutrients play a role, while verbal intelligence mainly reflects education and experience.

Healthy eating habits

The first symptoms of a marginal deficiency of a micronutrient are often psychological in nature. Children grow quickly, their metabolism is fast and there are high demands on their enzymes. Children often do not eat enough fresh fruit and vegetables. A supplement is necessary to prevent marginal deficiencies and ensure the optimal functioning of the nervous system (psychological development, memory, concentration, state of mind and intelligence) and the endocrine system (responsible for constant blood sugar levels, growth, thyroid function and development of the urogenital system).

It is important for children between the ages of two and 12 to learn healthy eating habits and to avoid refined sugar, white flour and greasy junk foods with a high fat content as much as possible. Children often enjoy being involved in planning their meals. From an early age teach them the principles of good nutrition and let them prepare the food themselves. Most children will understand and co-operate if they know why they must eat healthily. Children are more open to persuasion while they are still young. However, when they become a little more 'independent' between the ages of seven and 12 and develop their own likes and dislikes, they still usually eat the right kinds of food. If you just leave them and quietly observe what they eat over the course of a week or two, they will surprise you. You will be amazed at how healthy they eat when there is no pressure – and no parental eye watching their every action.

Never change mealtimes into unhappy stressful experiences. Children have an inherent motivation to eat, but their physiology is different. They master eating skills in the same way as other skills. They will naturally choose a variety of foods, not always on one day or exactly what their parents want them to eat. Children have a sensory-specific saturation level; they taste the food and eat just enough and of the right kinds. Adults often suppress or ignore the saturation stimulus and eat to satisfy cravings, for sociability or because food is good for you. We then force our children to eat the way we do by offering them desert or other rewards if they finish all their food.

The best thing for parents to do is to offer a variety of attractive, wholesome food in pleasant and comfortable surroundings and act positively. Children like a structured environment.

The most common nutrition problems during childhood are obesity and iron deficiency, not starvation. Even if there is a family history of cardiovascular disease and atherosclerosis, don't eliminate all fats. Avoid saturated fats and concentrate on low-fat milk, lean meat and mono- and polyunsaturated fats such as olive oil, flax oil, canola oil and grape seed oil. Stick to fresh fruit and vegetables, wholegrain products, seeds, nuts and pulses. Give your children a supplement combination for the cardiovascular system containing calcium and magnesium and the essential fatty acids. (Consult Chapters 7, 9 and 10.)

A good breakfast of hot oatmeal porridge or wholewheat cereal ensures constant blood glucose levels for improved concentration. Pack a nutritious lunch box with interesting sandwiches, pieces of raw vegetables and fruit or dried fruit and yoghurt to tempt their taste buds at break. Set a good example at home and remember that girls in particular soon pick up their mother's concerns about body mass and size. Don't overestimate your children's needs for food. A child's appetite depends on the rate at which they are growing and their activities – if you leave them alone, they will listen to the needs of their body. This is a natural instinct which many adults either suppress or forget. If adults also learned to tune in to their body more and listen to when the body needs food and exactly what it needs, there would be less concern with ideal body shapes and eating habits would be much healthier.

Exercise is important for all children and teenagers. The human body has developed to be physically active. The lifestyle of a lazy couch potato is bad for muscle development and state of mind.

A good nutritional supplement guarantees the children's needs and mothers can console themselves that the children have at least taken their daily health insurance in the form of micronutrients. Younger children prefer to take pills that they can chew, while older children can usually swallow the pills with water. Beware of sugar coated ("smartie") pills: the sugar coating process may destroy most of the pill's content! A general guideline for children under ten is half the adult dose.

Poor concentration and attention deficit hyperactivity disorder (ADHD)

About 5-10 per cent of schoolgoing children suffer from various degrees of poor concentration. It is four to six times more common in boys than girls. The main theory is that it is caused by a chemical imbalance in the concentration centre of the brain. The condition can improve considerably and even be cured through healthy eating habits with regular, small, wholesome meals to keep the blood glucose levels constant (low blood glucose increases hyperactivity and leads to poor concentration). In addition take essential fatty acids (for the deficiency of delta-6 desaturase), a supplement for the nervous system with chromium (200 micrograms), vanadium (50 micrograms) and molybdenum (200 micrograms) to keep blood sugar levels constant, calcium, magnesium and the amino acid taurine every day. Regular exercise is also important to channel the energy. Meditation and other relaxation techniques bring about a marked improvement in the ability to concentrate and quality of life. (Consult Chapters 9 and 10.)

In children with attention deficit hyperactivity disorder (ADHD) the immune system is often functioning below par. These children get a lot of infections and allergies, which aggravate the symptoms of hyperactivity. Taking antibiotics or other pharmaceutical medication aggravates the problem.

ADHD has become a fashionable diagnosis and it is made far too easily and quickly. The child's whole physical and psychological profile must be evaluated by a team of experts, including a medical doctor, a child psychologist, a speech therapist and eye specialist before the diagnosis can be made. Several disorders may seem like attention deficit. First eliminate hearing, speech and visual problems. Disturbed sleep is common in young children and can lead to symptoms of ADHD. Then eliminate petit mal (absency attacks) epileptic seizures. In older children you have to consider drug abuse, which can cause slowness and memory disorders. Depression, anxiety, tension and adapting to a new school or a new environment are often incorrectly diagnosed as attention deficit.

ADHD has a strong psychological component: food intolerance, allergy, micronutrient deficiency, infections, genetic factors, lead and other toxic metals, and psychological factors all play a role in the syndrome. Prescribing Ritalin for this is not going to work. Try an elimination diet. Supplements can often reduce or solve a dietary problem. My experience and that of other practitioners clearly show that the correct supplements, used together with stress management techniques, are extremely successful.

Daily supplementation

A good daily supplement (perhaps two or three products) for ADHD, attention deficit, poor concentration and memory, and for use during times of extra need such as exams and tests, will include the following (approximate amounts – the dose can be increased if the problem is serious):

- Vitamin C, 400 mg in two divided doses; the evening dose together with a calcium and magnesium supplement
- Vitamins B1-B5, about 20-25 mg of each
- Vitamin B12, 25 micrograms
- Folic acid, 400 micrograms
- Calcium, 500-600 mg
- Magnesium, 250-300 mg
- Zinc, 15 mg
- Inositol, 50 mg
- Choline, 50 mg
- Chromium, 100 micrograms
- Vanadium, 50 micrograms

- Molybdenum, 100 micrograms
- L-glutamine, 250 mg
- L-taurine, 250 mg
- Glycine, 250 mg
- Evening primrose oil, 1 000-2 000 mg
- Salmon oil, 600-1 500 mg

Many young children suffer from middle-ear infection, hyperactivity or both. The usual treatment includes antibiotics and grommets. The broad spectrum antibiotic destroys both the beneficial and the harmful bacteria. Research has shown that more than 75 per cent of middle-ear infections are caused by a virus and that antibiotics are ineffective as treatment. Taking antibiotics only leads to fungal infections (thrush or candida). Studies at the University of Colorado's Health Science Centre and the Yeshiva Medical School in New York have shown that children with recurring ear infections are three and a half times more prone to hyperactivity. Overproduction of Candida albicans may well be the common factor. The fungus secretes toxins which weaken the immune system and induce more infections. Candida can also cause irritation of the nervous system.

Try to put such a child on a natural alternative to antibiotics for a few weeks (consult Chapter 13), *Lactobacillus acidophilus* or *Bifidobacterium bifidus,* a supplement for the respiratory system and wholesome food, including live yoghurt cultures. In addition take essential fatty acids and a calcium and magnesium supplement and see what happens. This regime should work for any child with recurring infections.

Children with hyperactivity often have allergies as well. The culprits are usually milk, wheat, chocolate, eggs and cereals. Sugar can also aggravate the condition. Children who have sugar-sensitive symptoms of hyperactivity may have an underlying candida infection.

Allergies

Allergies are very common in the childhood years. To mention a few of the many factors involved – genetic tendency, pollution and smoking, toxins in food, tension (always look for signs of stress in children), marginal vitamin deficiencies and antibiotic abuse. Atopy (from the Greek for "difference"), the tendency to develop some form of allergic reaction, is often inherited, but the particular manifestation, including asthma, runny nose, eczema, nettle-rash (hives) and hay fever, is not necessarily hereditary.

An allergic reaction is in effect an antigen-antibody reaction. Anything that the body does not recognize as its own is seen as foreign and regarded as an antigen. The immune system produces antibodies to fight against the strange invaders The antibodies incite the white blood cells to become involved in the battle. These white blood cells, particularly the mast cells and eosinophils, secrete substances to get rid of the antigens. These substances cause changes in blood flow, muscle operation and mucous production. The body excretes the antigens through sneezing, coughing, nose-blowing, tears, perspiration, stools and breaking out in a skin rash.

The immune system produces antigens in various parts of the body to implement protection at strategic places. Cells in the mucous lining of the respiratory tract and digestive canal produce an antibody known as immunoglobulin E (IgE). Threatening antigens such as viruses and bacteria which enter the body through the airways or digestive tract activate the IgE. This leads to a cascade of inflammatory reactions to get rid of the antigens.

People who suffer from allergies have an overactive antigen-antibody reaction. Even harmless substances such as house mite, pollen, animal hair or wheat set off a reaction. In such a situation the antigen is called an allergen. Allergies can develop at any stage. Some babies get atopic skin changes when they aren't even two months old!

The treatment of allergies includes avoiding the allergen where possible. There are also sensitisation procedures in which the patient is exposed to small amounts of the allergen at regular intervals. Over a few weeks the dose is gradually increased. This sometimes helps to prevent the allergy (especially allergies to house mite and some grasses). The immune system gradually gets used to the allergen, but it is an expensive and drawn-out process (the course can take up to two years) and children do not like injections.

Antihistamines are another option. They interfere with the secretion of histamine by the mast cells in order to suppress the sneezing, congestion, itching and nettle rash. However, antihistamines can cause side effects that are often worse than the original symptoms. These include drowsiness, weakness, sluggishness, dry mouth, upset stomach and changes in the passing of stools. Expectorants, corticosteroids and nebulisers used to treat asthma also have side effects.

Conventional medicine focuses on treating the symptoms and suppressing the antigen-antibody reaction. The more natural treatment supports the immune system and reduces the overreaction. This is done in the following ways:

- Breastfeeding: Mother's milk until the baby is six months old or older is excellent for the prevention of allergies.
- Good wholesome nutrition: Avoid allergens, too much sugar and preservatives. Eat fresh fruit and vegetables, fish, etc.
- Food supplements: Essential fatty acids; antioxidants such as vitamins A, C and E, selenium, zinc and copper; calcium and magnesium; methyl sulphonyl methane (100 mg a day), a natural antihistamine; medicinal herbs; local application of herbs such as calendula, aloe vera and camomile; oatmeal porridge to calm the nerves and homeopathic remedies. (Consult the relevant chapters.)
- Stress management techniques: Good examples are meditation and progressive muscular relaxation. Meditation is a technique that can be used very effectively for children from the age of five until the teenage years and beyond to treat numerous psychological, allergic, concentration and self-image problems. (Consult Chapters 1, 2, 3, 9, 10, 11, 12, 13, 14 and 20.)

There is often confusion between the terms food allergy and food intolerance. A food allergy is an allergic reaction to certain foods, usually proteins. An immune reaction causes an abnormally high level of immunoglobulin E.

A food intolerance does not involve the immune system. It involves foods that produce drug related activities in the body. Examples include reactions from tomatoes and pineapple, bacterial toxins and infections, enzyme deficiencies (such as lactose) and synthetic additives such as tartrazine and sulphites.

General food intolerances are caused by sulphites in wine or reheated vegetables (hot flushes, congestion of the respiratory tract, low blood pressure), monosodium glutamate (MSG) in Chinese food (hypertension, perspiration, vomiting, headache, increased pressure in the face), tartrazine in yellow food colouring (congestion of the respiratory tract, itching, flushed skin) and as tyramine found in matured foods such as ripened cheese (hypertension when monoamine oxidase inhibitors are used for depression).

Acne

Acne can lead to a lot of unhappiness. It is a common problem encountered during the already difficult, sensitive, hormone-charged teenage years. Developing a positive self-image from an early age, stress management techniques, a healthy diet, drinking lots of water (eight glasses a day), regular exercise and supplements will go a long way towards improving and clearing acne.

Try using a cream or gel containing vitamins A, C and E on the skin. You can apply a gel containing aloe vera, calendula and arnica to active blemishes and an infected skin. You can also use a mask of marine algae extract with calendula, rosemary, eucalyptus oil, panthenol (a form of vitamin B5 that is good for the skin), jojoba oil and avocado oil twice a week on the skin. If the pimples are infected, apply topically and drink a natural 'antibiotic' mixture of herbs. (Consult Chapter 13.)

Remember to use the correct moisturiser on the skin morning and evening. Teenagers with acne often think their skin is too oily for a moisturiser and that moisturiser will exacerbate the condition. Quite the contrary – the less moisture your skin gets, the more irritated it becomes and the acne problem is aggravated.

Take the following daily supplements

- An antioxidant and multivitamin combination with the usual ingredients, but including high doses of vitamin A (10 000-15 000 IU or 3-4,5 mg of RE activity until the acne is under control and then 5 000-10 000 IU or 1,5-3 mg of RE activity), vitamin C (1 000-2 000 mg in divided doses), bioflavonoids (200 mg), vitamin E (200-400 IU), selenium (100 micrograms), zinc (30 mg), copper (2 mg), vanadium (100 micrograms), chromium (200 micrograms) and then as previously discussed.
- Calcium and magnesium as discussed.
- Essential fatty acids as discussed.
- Amino acids, especially those containing sulphur such as L-cysteine, N-acetyl-L-cysteine, methionine (250 mg of each) which are important for the functioning of the skin and as antioxidants. (Consult Chapter 5 on antioxidants.) Tyrosine (250 mg) supports thyroid function and plays a role in the pigmentation of skin and hair. (Consult Chapter 20 on the skin.)

Guidelines for supplements for healthy babies, children and teenagers

Remember that the quantity of each supplement is not as important as the combination of all of them together. Try a sugar-free, natural supplement that is sweetened with honey or fruit sugar – avoid the cheap, synthetic, sugar-coated ('smartie') supplements. The sugar-coating process destroys most of the vitamin and mineral content. If possible, take supplements where the minerals are in an amino acid chelation or food form.

1 Antioxidant and multivitamin supplement

The following is simply a general recommendation for healthy children to remain healthy. Consult the relevant chapter if your child suffers from a particular systemic problem. Use supplements as discussed in the chapter. For example, cases of respiratory tract allergies and respiratory tract infections such as tonsillitis and middle-ear infection are discussed in Chapter 14 on the respiratory system.

	Birth-2 years	3-11 years	12-18 years
Vitamin A	1 500 IU (455 µg or 0,5 mg RE activity)	2 500 IU (757 µg or 1 mg RE activity)	5 000 IU (1 515 µg or 1,5 mg RE activity)
Beta carotene (and mixed carotenes)	1 000 IU (1 mg)	2 000 IU (2 mg)	15 000 IU (10 mg)
Vitamin E	25 IU (24 mg)	50 IU (47 mg)	100 IU (83 mg)
Selenium	30 µg	50 µg	100 µg
Vitamin C	60 mg	150 mg	300 mg
Vitamin B1	0,5 mg	1 mg	2 mg
Vitamin B2	0,5 mg	1 mg	2 mg
Vitamin B3	7 mg	10 mg	20 mg
Vitamin B5	3 mg	4 mg	10 mg
Vitamin B6	1 mg	1,5 mg	3 mg
Vitamin B12	2 µg	5 µg	10 µg
Folic acid	60 µg	250 µg	400 µg
Biotin	30 µg	100 µg	200 µg
Chromium	60 µg	100 µg	200 µg
Copper	1 mg	1,5 mg	2 mg
Iron	5 mg	10 mg	15 mg
Manganese	1 mg	2 mg	5 mg
Molybdenum	30 µg	30 µg	30 µg
Potassium	0,7 mg	1 mg	2 mg
Zinc	4 mg	8 mg	10 mg

2 Calcium and magnesium supplement

(Always take it at night to improve the sleeping pattern)

	Birth-2 years	3-11 years	12-18 years
Calcium	200 mg	400 mg	600 mg
Magnesium	100 mg	200 mg	300 mg
Vitamin D	100 IU	100 IU	100 IU
Vitamin C	60-100 mg	60-100 mg	60-100 mg

3 Essential fatty acids

The following is simply a recommendation. Many supplements available on the market contain omega-3 and omega-6 fatty acids – just make sure that the supplement contains both.

	Birth-2 years	3-11 years	12-18 years
Evening primrose oil	500 mg	1 000 mg	1 000 mg
Salmon oil	300 mg	700 mg	700 mg

15.3 Treating childhood fevers

Most parents are unable to decide when to take a child to the doctor or when to try natural remedies first. Even experienced parents panic when their little ones get sick. Feelings of guilt come to the surface: a working mother, having to leave children at home alone, just deserts, neglect, etc. (Sounds familiar?) We look anxiously at the strange symptoms and wonder if it is too soon – or too late – to call the doctor.

Tips for parents

1 A natural phenomenon

All children get sick. This is a natural part of growing up and essential to obtain immunity. As children get older, they get fewer infections if the immune system has had the chance to develop a broad resistance to various viruses and bacteria. Abuse of antibiotics prevents the natural process of building up resistance. Always try the natural alternatives first (consult the relevant chapter) and try to restore the function of the relevant system with the right supplements (usually the respiratory system – consult Chapter 14). If there is no improvement after three to four days or if the condition gets worse, consult a doctor. That's what they're there for. Explain that you have used supplements. In most cases further medication will not be necessary. Recent research has shown that viral infections seems to be the cause in more than 75 per cent of cases even of middle-ear infection in children. Antibiotics are thus contraindicated. The doctor will examine for meningitis, appendicitis, tonsillitis and middle-ear infection and follow up as required.

2 Fever

Fever or an increased body temperature is the body's natural reaction to any kind of infection. Fever stimulates the immune system and sets it in motion. Fever is not a disease. If the temperature is brought down too quickly, it confuses the natural immune reaction and can ultimately delay the recovery process. The average body temperature is 37 degrees Celsius, but it varies from hour to hour and between adults and children. Factors that can increase a child's body temperature are a large meal, hot drinks, exposure to the sun, a fit of crying and exercise.

Medicines that bring down the fever too drastically can make the disease worse by curbing the capacity of the white blood cells to recognise a foreign invader. The linking of the antigen (foreign invader) to the antibody on the white blood cell membrane sends a chemical message to the hypothalamus in the brain. The hypothalamus increases the body temperature, activating more white blood cells and suppressing the multiplication and growth of viruses and bacteria.

If your child has a fever, but is calm and peaceful, leave him or her to sleep, lie or sit quietly as he or she prefers. However, if the child is restless and irritable, or in pain, give him a fever-reducing, anti-inflammatory painkiller containing ibuprofen, codeine and paracetamol. Let them lie quietly, give them plenty of fluids and relax.

Children with high temperatures seldom get brain damage. Fever is seldom a cause of death in a child. Fever convulsions are a disturbing and anxiety provoking experience for parents and children, but if a child is protected from physical harm, there is little damage and certainly no brain damage. Sponge the child with cool water or put the child in a cool bath. This, together with a tranquilliser (for parent and child) will soon bring an end to the convulsion. Fever convulsions are actually extremely rare.

Don't take a child's temperature too often. Never wake a sleeping child to take their temperature. This only makes the situation worse.

Fever does not necessarily mean bed rest. Let a child sleep as much as they want to, but don't force the issue. Children can stay at home quietly, read or watch television.

Consult your doctor if the temperature is 38 degrees Celsius, but the child is weak, listless and sleeps for too long; under the age of three months with a temperature of more than 37,9 degrees; three to six months with a temperature of more than 38,3 degrees; older than six months with a temperature of 39,4 degrees and if a temperature of 38,3 degrees lasts for longer than three days. Seek advice if the fever is associated with severe headache, coughing up of blood, severe irritability, vomiting, sever diarrhoea, severe skin rash and blood in the stools.

3 Hints for home nursing

(These tips work well for older children and fathers too - mothers don't get sick!)

- Give plenty of fluids to prevent dehydration as a result of fever and to keep the mucous liquid.
- Let them nibble bits of fruit and vegetables, cut into strips or slices. (Make shapes of clowns, cats, etc. – creative activity will distract your attention from your anxious worrying thoughts.) Give yoghurt and nutritious soup.
- Sponge down with lukewarm or cold water.
- Increase the intake of vitamin C, calcium and bioflavonoids until the condition improves and then return to the maintenance dose.
- Give medicinal herbs that support the immune system, destroy viruses and bacteria and have anti-inflammatory and fever-reducing properties and will dry up the mucous gently: Echinacea, golden

seal, garlic, milk thistle, yarrow, lime blossom, camomile and astragalus.

Don't get into a panic – that will just upset the child more. Remember that the body has a wonderful and efficient immune system to protect itself. It just needs a bit of TLC (tender, loving care) occasionally.

15.4 Treating herpes infections

This group of viruses is a common source of infection in human beings. It can vary from troublesome cold sores to glandular fever. As a group the herpes viruses are very infectious and can lie dormant in the body for long periods and break out as soon as the immune system is stressed. They cannot be treated with conventional medication. The most common herpes virus infections are cold sores, chicken pox, shingles, Epstein-Barr virus, cytomegalovirus and genital herpes.

Factors that can overload the immune system include disease, injury, emotional upsets, poor nutrition, too much exposure to sun and even menstruation. These may lead to outbreaks of herpes infections. The active herpes sores can allow other organisms to penetrate the body that would then lead to secondary infections.

Natural methods of treatment support the immune system, fight the herpes virus and provide pain relief. Follow these tips:

● Increase the intake of the amino acid L-lysine (500-2 000 mg a day on an empty stomach). Lysine supplements accelerate recovery and prevent recurrence of herpes infections. Lysine antagonises arginine which promotes herpes growth.
● Avoid processed foods, sugar, stimulants such as coffee, cola and chocolate, which put a greater burden on the immune system. Eliminate food with a high acid content: vinegar, citrus fruits and tomatoes. Limit salt intake. Milk and dairy products, seeds, nuts, peas and chocolate are high in arginine and should also be restricted during outbreaks.
● Medicinal herbs (as discussed in Chapter 13 on natural alternatives to antibiotics) can be taken internally and applied to the sores. A mixture of sage, Echinacea, aloe vera, arnica and calendula can be applied to mouth ulcers for quick relief.
● Vitamins and minerals support the immune system. Concentrate on

vitamin C (2 000 mg in divided doses during infection), vitamin E, B-complex vitamins and a zinc-amino acid combination (30 mg during infection).

● The sulphate polysaccharide content in red marine algae stimulates the antiviral reaction of the immune system by activating lymphocyte production which specifically fights viruses.

● Creams or gels containing aloe vera, calendula, golden seal powder (hydrastis), camomile and arnica can be applied locally for rapid relief. Repeat as required. A hot bath, with black tea leaves in it, also brings relief.

15.5 A natural first aid kit

It's wonderful to go on holiday! If you know that you can deal with upset stomachs, insect bites and infection, you will enjoy the break so much more. Medicinal herbs can be used to gently heal most minor accidents, tummy upsets and skin abrations. However, broken bones and serious infections need a doctor's attention.

Take herbal tinctures along with you. They are in concentrated form, immediately ready for use and small doses are sufficient.

● Jet lag can be prevented by using Siberian ginseng. This herbal remedy is an adaptogen that protects the body from the stress of long hours in the air and moving through different time zones. It improves intellectual alertness and job performance and enables the body to tolerate exhaustion, heat and noise. Use one dropper full of tincture or two capsules three times a day for two days before your departure. Stop taking it as soon as you reach your destination. You can also use a mixture of ginseng and hawthorn.

  Melatonin (3-6 mg two hours before bedtime) is also of value. It is a hormone produced by the pineal gland that regulates our day and night rhythm. However, it is not easily obtainable in South Africa. It is also an antioxidant, an anti-ageing substance and increases the production of serotonin. It relieves depression and seasonal affective disorder (SAD). (Consult Chapters 5 and 12.)

● Cuts, scrapes, bruises and insect bites can be treated with a mixture of Echinacea, golden seal, tea tree oil, aloe vera, calendula and camomile.

● An upset stomach can be treated with a tincture of dandelion, peppermint or camomile, three times a day. Ginger and *Ginkgo biloba* are good for motion sickness and psyllium works well for diarrhoea and chronic constipation. Take them with plenty of water. Take two teaspoons of the seed or one teaspoon of the bark, in water, twice a day.

● For sprained and pulled muscles or ligaments the usual rules apply – rest, ice, damp cloths/bandages and raising the affected limb. Alleviate swelling by applying horse chestnut gel. This will also improve the inflammation. Arnica, camomile and aloe vera gels also work well.

● For colds, flu and bladder infections, consult chapter 14 on the respiratory system (see recipe on page 170) and Chapter 13 on natural alternatives to antibiotics. Always have a herbal mixture containing Echinacea, hydrastis, garlic, camomile and astralagus for emergencies. Remember that cranberry juice is good for bladder infections.

15.6 Natural preparation for surgery

However well we look after our health, most of us will have to go to hospital at some stage in our lives for specialist treatment, special tests or surgery. You can maintain your holistic lifestyle with stress management, good nutrition, good supplementation and mental preparation even while in hospital. The fear of the procedure and its consequences places a burden on your immune system. It is worthwhile preparing yourself. Find out about the procedure. Talk to the doctor, anaesthetist and nursing staff and find out as much as you can.

Ask the surgeon to explain what is going to be done with a sketch or drawing. Discuss the side effects of the procedure and the anaesthetic. Don't let the doctors frighten you – insist on proper explanations. You are entitled to them. If you are informed, most of your fears and worries will disappear.

Do exercises that keep the mind calm and focussed, such as yoga and relaxation exercises. Aromatherapy, massage and reflexology will also keep you calm and reduce postoperative shock and pain.

Strengthen your immune system before you go to hospital. This will reduce postoperative infections and help you to recover more quickly. Eat healthy, wholesome foods. Take a good antioxidant supplement. Take twice your normal dose for two weeks before the operation and continue for six weeks after the operation. Echinacea, astragalus (also an adaptogen), aloe vera and golden seal are good immunostimulants and prevent postoperative infections. Use a tissue oil containing vitamins A, C and E, avocado oil, jojoba oil and wheatgerm oil on the site where the doctors will operate to reduce the formation of scars and enable the wound to recover more quickly. Start this a month before the operation and continue until the wound has healed completely.

Herbal adaptogens support the adrenal glands and improve the body's resistance to the stress of an operation. (An adaptogen is a substance that has the capacity to improve the body's resistance to a stressor.) Adaptogens support the adrenal function. Examples include astragalus, liquorice root, Korean, American and Siberian ginseng, as well as Reishi and Maitaki mushrooms. If you suffer from uncontrolled high blood pressure, consult your doctor before taking ginseng.

Hypericum (St John's wort, *Hypericum perforatum*) protects the body from the harmful effects of x-rays and postoperative depression. Kelp (marine algae) is also good for preventing the body from absorbing too much radioactive matter. It also protects the thyroid gland.

Aloe vera, bromelain (pineapple enzyme), turmeric and cayenne pepper reduce inflammation and pain. Kava kava reduces anxiety and sleeplessness – as do valerian root and camomile. Components of these herbs have an affinity for the same receptors in the brain as the benzodiasepines, but these herbs reduce anxiety without the associated suppression of the nervous system caused by benzodiasepines, which can lead to depression. (A recipe for a good sleeping potion is given on page 153.)

Take one capsule of acidophilus or lactobacillus three times a day and one teaspoon of psyllium seed in a glass of water if you are prone to constipation.

For postoperative nausea take a tea made with fresh ginger root and camomile three times a day. Also take 50 mg of vitamin B6 morning and evening after meals.

16 Natural remedies for weight management

This book only touches on certain aspect of weight management and slimming. A complete discussion falls beyond the scope of this book, but the topic will be fully discussed in a later book on health and slimming.

The subject of weight management and obesity is often a sensitive issue. Women especially have their own ideas of ideal size and shape – often distorted and unrealistic. The media obsession with perfect figures lets many women think that they should look like models. Take comfort in the thought that if you looked like that or could look like that, you would also be on the magazine covers. Remember that you may also be transferring your body obsessions to your daughter. The other day I heard of a young woman who came across her three-year old posing in front of the mirror, tugging at her clothing, face puckered up angrily and saying, 'Oh no, too tight, just look at me! I've put on another five kilograms!'

The secret of weight management is that your body mass should be optimal for your health and wellbeing. Your personality, genetic composition and circumstances determine your ideal weight at a particular stage of your life. Most people in their 40s, and having produced a couple of children, would not want to look the way they did at 16. Eat healthy, wholesome food. Eat regularly. Exercise regularly. Take the correct supplements. Practise stress management, meditate, relax. Your health will benefit the most from a regimen of mainly fresh vegetables and fruit, nuts, seeds, pulses, unsaturated fatty acids and unrefined carbohydrates. The resultant loss of body mass, while not your primary objective, will be a well-deserved bonus!

Facts and myths

There are health risks associated with obesity (diabetes, varicose veins, hypertension, back and feet problems, certain forms of cancer, osteo-arthritis, gall stones and cardiovascular diseases), but the health of people whose body mass seesaws is at even greater risk (such as increased occurrence of osteoporosis at an early age and premature ageing). The eternal 5 kg down, 7 kg up, 10 kg down, 12 kg up is probably the most dangerous health risk when it comes to managing body mass. One factor common to all people who live a particularly long and healthy life is that their body mass remains fairly constant throughout their adult life, even if it is 5-10 kg more than the average recommended normal weight.

Most of our weight obsessions are founded in a deep dissatisfaction within ourselves – no diet will remedy this. Accept yourself as you are. Learn to love yourself and reinforce the feeling every day. Get up in the mornings, look at yourself in the mirror and say, 'Good morning, you beautiful thing, I love you!' Try it. The fact that you feel ridiculous the first few times shows you where your real problem lies. You'll be amazed at how this simple sentence can change your attitude to life and interpersonal relationships. No matter what your circumstances are or what has happened in your life, you must love yourself. The rest will follow in due course. By loving yourself and accepting yourself as you are, you are accepting other people as they are. Being critical of others is often a reflection of how we feel about ourselves.

Many problems with body weight are psychological in origin and set up a vicious cycle: you are overloaded or depressed, you console yourself by eating unhealthy food, despise yourself for it, feel more depressed, eat again, feel self-conscious about your size, don't want to go out, get lonely, eat more, and so it goes on. Try to identify the problem and do relaxation exercises whenever you are feeling negative. Focus your attention on something else and the need to put something into your mouth will pass.

Carbohydrates and fats increase the secretion of serotonin and endorphins (the neurotransmitters). If you have premenstrual cravings for sweet things, chocolate or fattening snacks, or if you are depressed or pregnant, choose low-fat or sugar-free carbohydrate options, eat dried or fresh fruit like raisins (one handful) and grapes (one bunch). One little chocolate (bite-size) is not going to make you put on a kilogram or slow down your weight loss. Eat one and enjoy it rather than suppressing a craving that will only make you eat a whole slab or even a box of chocolates after a while.

The craving for 'something but I don't know what' is often a need for water. Drink a glass or two the next time you have that feeling. It will certainly help and is good for your health. Anyone who wants to lose weight must drink plenty of water and see to it that their diet is rich in fibre. This improves the functioning of the colon and helps the body to get rid of excess water and toxins.

Fad diets and rigidly prescriptive diets don't work – in fact, they do a lot of damage. Your body goes into starvation mode and your metabolism virtually comes to a standstill. You lose a lot of water, which deceives you into thinking that you have lost 3 kg in two days. Then you start to lose muscle tissue and after about two weeks you start to break down fat. By that time you have already given up on the dreadful diet. After every fad diet the body stores as much fat as it can to make provision for the next famine period. This is how the human specie has survived. Your physiology does not know that it is not fashionable to look well-rounded and healthy. Hunger strikes do not work either. If you eat nothing all morning, by four in the afternoon your blood sugar has dropped alarmingly and you raid the pantry, the fridge (even the dog's bowl looks appealing) and you eat anything you can get hold of.

The only thing that works is to eat regular, small meals to ensure constant blood sugar levels and good nutrition. Take regular exercise in the form of walking, dancing or aerobic exercise three to five times a week with good food supplements to provide all the micronutrients you need and you will be healthy and slim. Choose an exercise you enjoy; otherwise you won't keep it up. If you are not in the habit of exercising, start slowly (ten minutes a day) and increase it gradually to 20 minutes every day or 30-60 minutes three to five times a week. Even by parking further away from the office or the shops, you will get a fair amount of exercise if you walk fast. Use the stairs instead of the lift. Before you start exercising, do some warming-up, stretching exercises to prevent muscle injury. Joining a walking group is a good idea - it is pleasant, cheap (you only need a pair of good walking shoes), people encourage one another and it is safe.

Food combining is also unnecessary – except when people have specific health problems if they eat certain foods such as curry or people who have ulcers or gastritis not eating tomatoes. If you combine vegetables and carbohydrates, you are taking in proteins as well. Most carbohydrates and all fruits also contain proteins. Our digestive tract is designed to handle all types of food. As soon as the food gets into your mouth, the digestive enzymes further down the alimentary tract are already secreted, even before the food gets there. These include the enzymes that break down the proteins, fats and carbohydrates into the basic amino acids, fatty acids, glycerol and glucose.

Food does not only have a material (physical) value; it also provides pleasure and fulfilment. It also forms an important part of our social structure. We derive emotional and mental benefits from the food we eat. Diets negate and suppress all these natural needs and convey the message to our mind and body that the only way to lose body weight is through punishing your body. The body reacts to this suppression by staging a general rebellion. This leads to excessive feelings of hunger, delayed metabolism and even disease processes.

The answer is balance. Learn to understand your body's needs – eat when your body tells you to and what it tells you to eat. It can take a while before you learn to interpret the signs correctly. Be patient. Don't berate or insult yourself. Examine yourself through prayer, meditation and relaxation techniques. This works.

Remember – you are what you eat. All the foods are broken down into basic molecules that are used again in the body to form substances such as neurotransmitters which determine your state of mind and emotions, to form the muscle and bone cells that operate your heart and skeleton and form every immune cell and all the hormones which control every function of your body and mind. The quality of every organ and system depends on the quality of each cell. This is determined by the quality of the food and supplements you take in and your mental condition. Always think of this when you nourish your body and soul physically, emotionally and mentally.

Micronutrients and supplements to support weight management

Use a good multivitamin and antioxidant combination with B-complex vitamins, a calcium and magnesium supplement and essential fatty acids to allow all systems to function optimally, ensuring optimal combustion of fats and delaying the ageing process (cell damage by free radicals, osteoporosis, mental degeneration).

Some micronutrients are effective in accelerating the metabolism a little, keeping the blood glucose levels constant and stimulating the satiety centre. Others help the body to excrete toxins and excess water as well as providing more energy. This is discussed briefly. Excessive body weight as a result of a 'glandular problem' is extremely rare. People who suffer from hypothyroidism (underactive thyroid gland) will also benefit from the following supplements:

- L-carnitine or acetyl-L-carnitine (500-1 000 mg a day on an empty stomach) is probably the best-known amino acid for reducing body mass. Research has shown that carnitine is very effective in weight management programs. Carnitine assists the mitochondria (power generators of the cell) to utilise fats for energy production. This improves the utilisation of fat for energy and makes stored fat available for conversion into energy. It is therefore effective for fat break down and improves metabolism. The action of carnitine is especially effective when combined with aerobic exercise such as walking, jogging, dancing and aerobics. Any exercise which requires oxygen and is done for a period longer than 20 minutes is aerobic. (The role of carnitine in the cardiovascular system and for people who participate in sport is discussed in Chapters 6 and 7.)

- L-phenyl alanine (500-1 000 mg a day on an empty stomach) increases the production of cholecystokinin, a compound that suppresses the appetite. Phenyl alanine is also a precursor of the neurotransmitters dopamine and noradrenaline that improves state of mind. Phenyl alanine also strengthens the other mood-enhancing chemicals, namely phenylethol alanine and the endorphins. It is often used in the treatment of depression and as a painkiller, especially in chronic pain. Phenyl alanine also improves mental alertness.

  Note that phenyl alanine should not be used by people who are suffering from phenylketonuria.

- L-tyrosine (500-1 000 mg a day on an empty stomach) is a precursor of dopamine, adrenalin and noradrenaline. Each of them is involved in the stress reaction and they soon become depleted during long periods of stress. L-tyrosine is used in the treatment of depression and mental exhaustion. Tyrosine improves the body's ability to handle the mental, psychological and physical implications of stress. Tyrosine is also needed for the production of the thyroid hormones and is valuable in treating hypothyroidism. This increases the metabolism and thereby reduces body mass and improves fat breakdown for energy.

- Taurine (500 mg a day on an empty stomach) is another amino acid that improves fat combustion and fat metabolism. It improves the secretion of bile and is thus used to treat stones in the gall bladder. Taurine is also effective in controlling hypertension and high cholesterol and is used to treat anxiety, tension, panic attacks, attention deficit and disturbed sleep.

- Chromium (about 200 micrograms a day) in an amino acid chelation or food form is of great value in weight loss because it ensures constant blood sugar levels and it reduces the craving for sweet things. Many cases of obesity may be due to a lack of chromium. A high sugar intake further lowers the chromium content of the body.

- Vanadium (about 75 micrograms a day) and molybdenum (about 30 micrograms a day) prevents atherosclerosis and assists glucose transfer into the cells.

- Choline (about 100 mg a day) and inositol (about 50 mg a day) are both B-complex vitamins that improve fat and cholesterol metabolism. Both are lipotrophic vitamins. This means that they improve fat utilisation by cells for energy production. Both support weight loss.

- Co-enzyme Q10 (about 30 mg a day in divided doses) improves the oxygen utilisation and energy metabolism of cells. It is a moderate metabolic stimulant and can encourage weight loss.

- Garcinia cambogia (in the form of hydroxycitric acid, 400 mg a day), a primary acid in the fruit and peel of the *Garcinia cambogia* plant, suppresses fat synthesis, reduces the production of LDL-cholesterol and triglycerides, suppresses appetite and increases the body's production of heat by means of thermogenesis. Thermogenesis promotes fat breakdown for the energy needed to maintain the increased heat production.

- Other medicinal herbs that can be of value in treating obesity and increasing the energy levels include the adaptogens such as the various ginsengs and the Reishi mushroom, ginger root to improve digestion, astragalus to get rid of excess water and support the immune system, kelp (marine algae, *Fucus vesiculosis*) to improve the excretion of toxins and to increase the metabolism by stimulating the thyroid hormone production, and camomile and peppermint to improve digestion. Chicory *(Cichorium intybus)* acts as a diuretic to get rid of excess fluid. (Consult Chapter 13 for more information on herbs.)

- Royal jelly contains key ingredients for more energy, mental alertness and a general feeling of wellbeing. It also improves the immunity and acts at cellular level to repair system functioning. It is rich in pantothenic acid (vitamin B5), an important vitamin for dealing with stress, insomnia and fatigue. It improves digestion and ensures healthy hair and nails.

- Betasitosterol is another plant product that shows potential for controlling weight and cholesterol. It is a plant sterol compound that attaches itself to the same receptors in the intestine as saturated fats and cholesterol. It thereby prevents the absorption of saturated fats and cholesterol. The betasitosterol itself is not absorbed, nor does it interfere with the digestion and absorption of essential nutrients, vitamins and minerals. It does not cause allergic reactions. It induces a natural feeling of satiety and reduces the appetite. The unabsorbed saturated (bad) fat is excreted in the stools. It can be safely used by children and diabetics.

Betasitosterol reduces fat and cholesterol absorption and serves as a natural lubricant for the colon. It reduces bloating, constipation and flatulence in the digestive system. It ensures more efficient excretion of waste material and protects the intestines against harmful toxins which may be a factor in cancer of the intestine and colon.

The dose depends on the amount of saturated fat you eat. This is the fat intake you need to reduce drastically in any case as part of a healthy eating pattern. If you eat salad with a little olive oil, you won't need to take betasitosterol. However, if you eat a greasy hamburger with chips, you will need to take three capsules of betasitosterol beforehand! This is not to say that you can eat the wrong things and then correct the damage by taking betasitosterol beforehand! It is a remedy to help you improve your general health by lowering cholesterol and relieving constipation – especially if you've been overdoing things. Take the capsules 30 minutes before meals with at least one glass of water.

- Fibre such as bran, psyllium, pectin and guar bean gum do not prevent fat absorption, they simply reduce the amount of time the food spends in the intestine by accelerating the passage of fat, cholesterol and carcinogens. Most of the fat is still absorbed. Fibre is an excellent tool for weight management, because it improves constipation, and assists the body in getting rid of toxins.

In conclusion

These are a few remedies you can try in your efforts to have a healthy, slim and fit figure. They are not intended as quick solutions to weight loss. They will simply help you maintain the discipline needed to establish a new lifestyle.

17 Micronutrients for the female urogenital system

Many of the problems that women have to deal with can be solved by making some lifestyle changes. The pace of life today places a heavy burden on women, many of whom find themselves having to juggle the demands of a household, a marriage, children's activities and a taxing career – either from home or an office. Quality of life is often set aside and the time that is so essential for relaxation, being quiet and catching one's breath is sacrificed. This causes enormous stress, fatigue, infections such as candida and problems such as premenstrual syndrome (PMS), infertility and a difficult menopause. (Consult Chapter 18 for more information on menopause.)

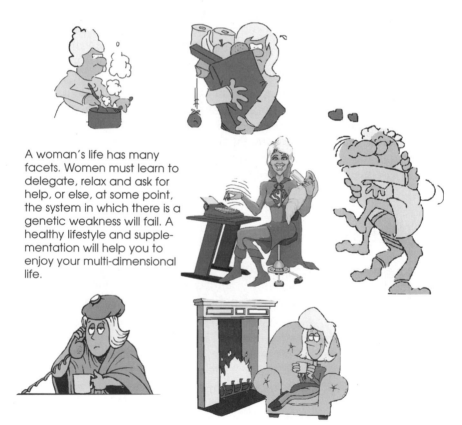

A woman's life has many facets. Women must learn to delegate, relax and ask for help, or else, at some point, the system in which there is a genetic weakness will fail. A healthy lifestyle and supplementation will help you to enjoy your multi-dimensional life.

Stress management, taking time for oneself each day (relaxation, meditation, prayer – time for self-reflection and objective assessment of the day's activities), moderate exercise, healthy eating habits and correct supplementation with micronutrients will help to alleviate almost all 'female' complaints.

Everything starts with a good multivitamin and antioxidant combination, specifically directed to repair the function and balance of the female hormones. Specific ingredients that focus on the treatment of any disorder of the female urogenital system are briefly discussed.

From the teenage years onwards, for the rest of her life, every woman should take daily supplements of calcium and magnesium and essential fatty acids containing omega-3 and omega-6 fatty acids. It is never too late to start. Good comprehensive combinations are more important than the quantities of the individual ingredients.

Vitamins

- Vitamin A (5 000-10 000 IU or 1 515-3 030 micrograms of or 1,5-3 mg of RE or vitamin A activity a day) ensure rapid recovery of the mucous lining of the womb after menstruation, as well as the recovery of the mucosa of the whole urinary tract and genital system after infections such as candida and cystitis (bladder infection) and injury such as Caesarian section, birth and hysterectomy. Vitamin A protects the mucous layers against the damage from free radicals and delays the ageing of the skin. It also protects the female urogenital system from cancer of the cervix and the uterus (womb). Vitamin A is used in the treatment of PMS and fibrocystic breast disease (fibroadenosis or benign breast lumps, especially painful, swollen and tender before menstruation). Take vitamin A together with 25 000 IU (25 mg) of beta and other carotenes for serious acne, associated with PMS. Choline and inositol (100 mg of each a day) help to provide nutrients for the skin. Zinc (20 mg a day) is also good for acne.
- Beta carotene and other carotenoids (15 000-25 000 IU or 10-15 mg a day) form vitamin A as required and act as antioxidants themselves. This reduces acne and other skin problems and is im-portant for the prevention of breast cancer and other cancers of the urogenital system.
- Vitamin C (1 000-2 000 mg a day in divided doses) is an important

antioxidant that delays ageing. It helps to reduce hot flushes and accelerates tissue repair. It is an essential vitamin for every woman. (Consult Chapter 5 on antioxidants.)

- Vitamin E (400 IU or 332 mg a day) protects sensitive tissue such as the urogenital system and skin against the damage from free radicals and supports the biological activity of vitamin A. Vitamin E prevents tissue degeneration, thereby preventing premature ageing and promoting longevity. It is often used to treat PMS, fibroadenosis, dysmenorrhoea (painful menstruation) and menopausal symptoms, especially hot flushes. It prevents blood clotting – particularly important in the prevention and treatment of heart attacks, deep vein thrombosis and pulmonary embolism. Vitamin E prevents degeneration of tissue in varicose veins. Vitamin E can curb the sweet craving experienced by so many premenstrual women. Chromium 200 micrograms), vitamin B1 (100 mg), B6 (200 mg) and other B-complex vitamins can also be used for this purpose.

- Vitamin B1 (thiamine, 100-150 mg a day) alleviates most symptoms of PMS, namely depression, fatigue, irritability, dejection, fluid retention, tension, anxiety and sweet cravings.

- Vitamin B2 (50 mg a day) is used to treat PMS, especially tension and fatigue. It supports cellular respiration and improves the oxygen utilisation of all cells. Riboflavin ensures normal cell growth and recovery after damage.

- Vitamin B3 (50 mg a day) is important for the formation of oestrogen and progesterone. It is used to supplement the body's store of energy and is valuable in treating fatigue, irritability, depression and anxiety – all symptoms of PMS. Niacin is prescribed for the treatment of low blood sugar (hypoglycaemia), migraine and acne. It also improves the libido.

- Vitamin B6 (100-200 mg a day) is generally used in the treatment of PMS symptoms. It reduces fluid retention and helps for painful, sore breasts. Vitamin B6 is often used to treat moodiness, depression, low libido, fatigue, anxiety and tension. All women who are on contraceptive medication or hormone replacement therapy should take supplementary pyridoxine.

- Folic acid (400 micrograms a day) is responsible for the maturation of red blood cells and assists in the break down and utilisation of proteins in the body. It is essential for the formation of RNA and DNA in the cell nucleus and plays a fundamental role in the growth and reproduction of cells. Supplements are necessary for women who are pregnant or breastfeeding, to prevent dysplasia, cancer of the cervix, osteoporosis, for dementia (Alzheimer's disease) and to treat megaloblastic anaemia (together with vitamin B12).

● Vitamin B12 (100 micrograms a day) is responsible for the production of red blood cells, cell growth and reproduction and the metabolism of nerve tissue. Cobalamin is also known as the energy and longevity vitamin because it increases energy levels and improves the activity of the nervous system. Vitamin B12 is often used in the treatment of fatigue, pernicious anaemia, delayed growth in children, neuralgia, depression, irritability, insomnia, anxiety, poor memory, osteoporosis and arthritis.

Minerals

● Calcium (600-900 mg a day in an amino acid chelation or food form) is used to treat menstrual cramps, irritability, anxiety, leg cramps, insomnia and osteoporosis.

● Magnesium (500-1 000 mg a day) is very effective for treating PMS, painful menstruation, irritability, anxiety and depression.

● Iron (15 mg a day in an amino acid chelation or food form) is recommended for all women who are still menstruating. Supplements are also essential during pregnancy and breastfeeding.

● Zinc (20 mg a day) is important for the treatment of skin complaints and for maintaining the function of the urogenital system.

● Iodine (300 micrograms a day) is not really needed as a supplement, except if you suffer from hypothyroidism (underactive thyroid). Iodine is essential in the formation of the thyroid hormones that regulate our metabolism. Thyroid hormones are responsible for the actual function, respiration, growth and development of every cell in the body. It affects every bodily function. It is important for cell propagation, normal state of mind, the functions of vitamin A, healthy hair and nails, and the prevention of cancer of the breast, ovaries and uterus.

Amino acids

L-methionine (500 mg a day on an empty stomach) is an amino acid that can be of value in treating PMS. It can assist in the removal of excess oestrogen from the body. High oestrogen levels are implicated in PMS (especially anxiety and irritability). The contraceptive pill and hormone replacement therapy produce very high levels of oestrogen in the body which the liver is not always able to handle and the oestrogen accumulates in the body. This leads to the increased synthesis of fats (building up of fat tissue) which can restrict the liver function even further. Methionine and vitamin B6 are very effective in treating the side effects of the contraceptive pill and hormone replacement therapy.

Essential fatty acids

Essential fatty acids are very important in the treatment of PMS, painful menstruation, depression and tension. They are strongly recommended for the maintenance of all the functions of the female urogenital system.

Medicinal herbs

- Angelica (*Angelica sinensis* or dong quai, two capsules or tea twice a day) is a Chinese herbal remedy that has been used for centuries to keep the female urogenital system in balance. It is a general tonic for the female system and is often prescribed in the West for painful menstruation, PMS, fatigue, menopausal symptoms and weakness after childbirth.
- Ginger root (2,5 ml of chopped fresh root in a glass of boiling water with honey or in food or two capsules twice a day) is a good way of improving blood circulation and counteracting fluid retention (PMS). It is anti-inflammatory and can be used for painful menstruation. Ginger also improves digestion.
- Parsley, asparagus, celery and cucumber work well for fluid retention.
- Liquorice root, with ginger in a tea, is generally effective for keeping the female urogenital system in balance.
- White willow bark *(Salix alba)* is the natural form of aspirin which is effective for painful menstruation because of its anti-inflammatory properties.

- Hawthorn berry *(Crateagus oxyacantha)* helps for menstrual cramps and low blood pressure associated with menstruation.
- Peony root improves vascular contraction to ensure the rapid recovery of the uterus after menstruation. It helps for menstrual cramps and restores the hormone balance in the female urogenital system.

Consult Chapter 18 on the menopause for other herbs that can be of value for the female urogenital system. Most of them will help for PMS and dysmenorrhoea.

Medicinal herbs that are often prescribed by herbalists for treating infertility in women include chaste tree berry *(Vitus agnus castus)*, dong quai, red clover blossom, liquorice root and Siberian ginseng. All these herbs either contain active ingredients which can stimulate hormone production or phyto-oestrogens that stimulate ovulation.

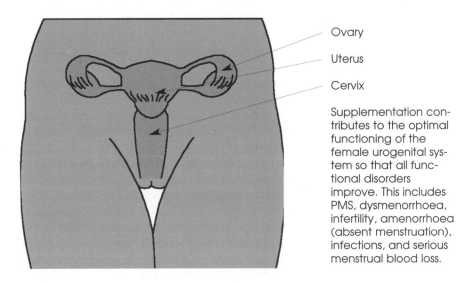

Ovary

Uterus

Cervix

Supplementation contributes to the optimal functioning of the female urogenital system so that all functional disorders improve. This includes PMS, dysmenorrhoea, infertility, amenorrhoea (absent menstruation), infections, and serious menstrual blood loss.

Natural treatment of candida infection

Candida albicans (white) is a fungus or yeast that is always present in the body. The growth of candida is controlled by the beneficial bacteria in the digestive tract and the female urogenital system.

The excessive use and abuse of antibiotics results in the uninhibited growth of candida. Unfortunately, antibiotics kill the good, harmless, beneficial bacteria along with those that cause disease. Candida then begins to proliferate because the natural growth control is no longer present. This causes thrush in babies and young children and candidiasis in adult women. Babies get thrush if their bottles are too much sterilised, which then destroys the good bacteria. Rinse dummies and bottles in water after removing them from the sterilising solution. Although it is mainly women who get candida infections, men can become infected. This is why partners should both be treated even if only the one has the infection – otherwise cross-infection takes place.

The contraceptive pill disturbs the normal hormone balance in the female urogenital system and can result in excessive growth of candida. Diabetics are also prone to candida infections (candida organisms like sugar). If you often have problems with candida, you should have a glucose tolerance test.

Symptoms

Candida can manifest in various ways:

- Chronic vaginal infections characterised by a thick white, crumbly, itchy discharge. This is often mistakenly regarded as the only symptom of candida infection.
- Infections in the mouth and the rest of the digestive tract with a white layer on the tongue, sore throat, painful and red mucosa in the mouth, anus, penis, skin, fingernails and toenails.
- Systemic infection on account of increased intestinal permeability that allows candida fungi to enter the bloodstream ('leaky gut' syndrome). This can cause diarrhoea, general fatigue, low libido, menstrual disorders, muscular pain, painful joints, headache, bloating, allergies, reduced immune function in chronic respiratory infections, depression and poor concentration. A conclusive diagnosis can only be made by undergoing specific tests (for example, a test for candida antibodies with IgG, IgM, IgA, as well as food tolerance tests, white blood cell count and a glucose tolerance test).

Treatment

First be sure that you do have a candida infection by going for a routine check-up and a vaginal smear. The natural remedies are directed at the improvement of general health and wellbeing. The following recommendations will benefit your health in any event:

- Avoid antibiotics as much as possible – take them only if it's really essential. If all contraceptive medications cause candidiasis, you will have to find another method of contraception. Corticosteroids and the medicines used to treat ulcers can also cause candida. Try other options under your doctor's supervision – your doctor should be aware of complementary therapies.
- Support the immune system with herbs such as Echinacea, golden seal *(Hydrastis canadensis)*, calendula and garlic. (Consult Chapter 13 on natural alternatives to antibiotics.) Most of these herbs will keep the fungal growth in check. Apply them to the affected area and take them orally. Tea tree oil and lavender oil are gentle enough to use on infected skin and the mucosa. Apply directly to the skin or put three drops of each on a vaginal tampon or sanitary towel. You can also add these oils to the bathwater (ten drops of each). Regular use should soon clear the problem. Capsules of *Lactobacillus acidophilus* or *Bifidobacterium bifidum* (two capsules twice a day) will also contribute to the regrowth of a normal bacterial population in the body thereby balancing the excessive growth of candida. These capsules can either be taken orally or opened up and made into a paste to apply directly into the vagina. Natural yoghurt can also be used as a douche. Mix natural yoghurt with 10 ml of apple vinegar, ten drops of tea tree oil and 10 ml of golden seal root extract (hydrastis); add the mixture to a hot bath and have a long soak.
- Avoid refined sugar, white flour, white rice, canned or processed foods, alcohol, fizzy drinks, coffee, fruit juices, bananas, grapes, fermented foods such as cheese, smoked fish, dairy products, honey and mushrooms for 30 days. If your symptoms improve, you will know that the problem is candida. In any event, you will feel much healthier, more energetic and lose a few kilograms as well.
- Don't wear tight-fitting underwear or clothing – avoid vaginal deodorants, soap, powder and perfume. Avoid underwear made from synthetic fabrics such as nylon. Wear cotton panties.
- Eat plenty of fresh fruit (exept for those mentioned) and vegetables,

natural unflavoured yoghurt, fibre-rich foods, brown rice, fresh fish, chicken, olive oil, oatmeal porridge and drink plenty of water.

● Take vitamin and mineral supplements and include them in your diet to support the immune system and the urogenital system.

– Vitamin A (10 000 IU or 3 030 micrograms or 3 mg of RE activity a day during the infection, then reduced to 5 000 IU a day).

– Vitamin C (2 000 mg a day in divided doses during the infection and then reduced to 1 000 mg a day).

– Vitamin E (400 IU or 332 mg a day) with 100 IU of selenium a day.

– Beta carotene, magnesium, calcium, B-complex vitamins, co-enzyme Q10, molybdenum, chromium and essential fatty acids (omega-3 and omega-6) will all contribute to curing and preventing candida infection.

– Bioflavonoids (Echinacea, garlic, quercetin, peppermint, camomile, rose hip, pawpaw, green pepper, broccoli and tomatoes are all rich in bioflavonoids).

– Zinc (15 mg a day).

● Stress management is essential in the treatment of candida infection. Chronic stress weakens the action of the immune system and aggravates the frequency and duration of the disease. Most people who have to cope with the burden of recurrent candida infection are psychologically, physically and emotionally taxed. Balance must be restored – not only in your intestinal flora but also in your life. Outbreaks of the disease are often connected with stress at work, changes in living circumstances and the eternal conflict between work, domestic chores and family life – the modern woman's dilemma! (Consult Chapters 1 and 2 on stress and stress management.)

Think of candida as a lesson that you have encountered that will teach and help you to restore balance in your body, emotions, mind and soul. A positive attitude will soon return you to the path towards health and wellbeing.

18 Menopause and hormone replacement therapy

Most women are aware from a very early age that women eventually have to go through menopause. A woman's ovaries can stop producing oestrogen and progesterone at any time – usually between the ages of 45 and 50 but it can vary between 40 and 55. However, the production of oestrogen in the body never stops completely and it is also produced in several other organs of the body. The initial symptoms of menopause can be attributed to the sudden decrease in the production of oestrogen and progesterone from the ovaries. The severity and duration of symptoms also depend on various other factors.

Men also experience symptoms of transition or change of life. However, the decrease in the production of testosterone is not as drastic as that of oestrogen and progesterone and it takes place more gradually.

Symptoms associated with menopause

- Irregular periods
- Hot flushes with night sweats, heart palpitations, nausea and anxiety
- Headaches
- Fluid retention with swelling and oedema
- Tender, painful breasts
- Lowered libido and vaginal dryness
- Insomnia (aggravated by hot flushes)
- Fatigue
- Muscle and joint aches and pains
- Irritability and impatience
- Emotional instability
- Depression
- Loss of short-term memory
- Lack of concentration

Most of the symptoms can be attributed to a progesterone deficiency, sleep deprivation and stress rather than an oestrogen deficiency. Remember that many factors play a role in the development, severity and duration of menopause. The change in hormone levels is only one of the factors. Heredity, general health, nutritional status, medication, lack of exercise, stressful events in your life (children leaving home, difficult teenagers, financial problems, marriage problems, looking after elderly parents) and your whole attitude to life all play their part. A woman's body can compensate for the decline in ovarian oestrogen production by increasing production in other organs (the adrenal glands, liver, fatty tissue and brain). It is mainly the increased emotional and nutritional demands that may put too great a burden on the body and mind. This can aggravate menopausal symptoms.

More than 300 types of tissue in the body contain receptors for oestrogen and progesterone. A marked decrease in the amount of oestrogen and progesterone from the main source (the ovaries) will clearly cause dramatic physical changes.

Symptoms of low oestrogen and progesterone

- Genital organs (vagina, vulva, uterus) – vaginal dryness, thin atrophied mucosa and skin, lowered libido, vaginal infections caused by pH change (acid content) in mucosa
- Urinary tract (kidneys, ureter, bladder, urethra) – incontinence, infections
- Breasts – tenderness, nodosity
- Skin – dryness, sensitivity
- Hair – dryness, hair loss
- Mucosa – dryness, airway infections, airway allergies, digestive problems
- Skeleton – osteoporosis
- Cardiovascular system – hypertension, high LDL-cholesterol, angina, heart attacks, stroke
- Pelvic muscles – poor muscle tone in bladder floor with stress incontinence (leakage of urine while laughing, coughing or exercising)
- Brain – depression, emotional instability

Like puberty, menopause causes dramatic changes in a woman's body. The process takes place over a period of one to five years, with menstrual periods becoming less frequent until they stop altogether.

**Many women do not even realise that
they're going through menopause.
Do not expect to get any symptoms.
You may be one of the lucky ones!**

Coping with menopausal symptoms

Remember that the natural approach to coping with menopause is geared towards making the process easier for women rather than stopping the natural process indefinitely. Research has shown that two thirds of women on prescription hormone replacement therapy (HRT) stop taking it after a year because of the side effects.

1 Positive attitude

The single most important factor in managing menopause is a positive attitude. Stress management techniques are essential, as well as coming to terms with the fact that you are getting older and entering a new phase in your life where you will have more time for yourself, your needs and your personal growth. It is a time of maturation and wisdom. Your reproductive role is over and you can contribute to the community and your family on a deeper level of wisdom and support.

2 Energy levels

Energy levels may be low during menopause. Try to get enough sleep. Take a morning or afternoon nap if you have trouble sleeping at night. Special foods that supply plenty of vitamins, minerals and energy include raw honey, red grapes with the pips, spirulina, *Rosa roxburghii*, Chlorella, brewer's yeast, molasses, lecithin and kelp (or marine algae).

3 Water

Drink plenty of water (at least eight glasses a day). Water keeps the body young and energetic, with all the biochemical reactions functioning at peak performance. Water also diminishes the cravings for sweet, salt or that indescribable 'something' we often feel like. These cravings often indicate a deficiency of fluids or water in the body.

4 Diet

Ensure that your diet contains fresh, wholesome food, including plenty of fruit and vegetables, wholegrain products, nuts, seeds and pulses. Oatmeal porridge is a good tonic – it provides fibre (roughage), lowers the LDL-cholesterol and contains many vitamins and minerals. Consume the recommended food throughout the day in six or eight small portions to prevent low blood sugar (hypoglycacmia), which aggravates menopausal symptoms.

Eat fish, poultry, eggs, dairy products, cold pressed olive, canola and linseed (flax) oil sparingly.

Avoid refined sugar, white flour, processed foods, processed meats, fried food, saturated (mainly animal) fat, preservatives and too much alcohol.

A diet with enough good quality protein of and plenty of B-complex vitamins will support the pituitary gland, which in turn controls the ovaries and the female hormone cycle. This slows down the onset of menopause. Note that women who are strict vegetarians with a very low cholesterol level tend to go through an earlier menopause. Remember that cholesterol can also be very important for the production of female hormones.

Eat foods that are rich in proteins such as fish, dairy products (low-fat yogurt and cottage cheese), eggs, wholegrain products, pulses, nuts and seeds every day.

Foods that contain the B-complex vitamins include green vegetables, wholegrain products, wheatgerm and yeast. Adequate levels of pantothenic acid (vitamin B5), choline and inositol support the adrenal glands and the pituitary gland.

Soya is a rich source of proteins, minerals, vitamins and natural phyto-oestrogens (from plants) that can compensate for the body's lowered production of oestrogen. These include soya beans, tofu and soya flour. Vegetarian cookery books contain many delicious recipes for tasty soya dishes. You can also mix soya flour with ordinary wholegrain flour. Two of the active ingredients in soya beans, daidzain and genistein, have various functions: they are effective against menopausal symptoms and as antioxidants they protect the body against premature ageing and many diseases such as cardiovascular disease, osteoporosis and cancer.

Linseed oil (flax oil) contains plenty of these plant oestrogens. Add the seeds to salads, sauces and sandwich spreads. A tablespoon of linseed in a glass of water is also good for constipation.

5 Calcium supplements

Calcium supplements are essential. It is better to prevent osteoporosis rather than to wait until there are signs of it. The body's minimum daily calcium requirement is 1200 mg, which is almost impossible to obtain through diet alone. Your supplement should also contain magnesium, vitamin D (150-400 IU a day), vitamin C (600-1 000 mg a day), boron (2-3 mg a day) and potassium (150 mg a day) to ensure optimum calcium absorption and bioavailability. Boron also elevates oestrogen levels naturally.

Women should start to use calcium supplements as early as possible, but it is never too late to start. Calcium and magnesium are involved in many functions in the body. Ensuring an additional daily supply prevents the body from taking it out of the bones. An adequate supplementation dose during menopause would be 900-1 000 mg of calcium a day and 450-500 mg of magnesium a day. The best way to absorb calcium and magnesium is to take it in an amino acid chelation (amino acids are the building blocks of proteins). This ensures optimal absorption in the intestinal tract and bioavailability to the cells. Other good calcium compounds are carbonate or citrate form.

Foods rich in calcium that help to ensure strong bones include fish, leafy greens, wholegrain products and dairy products such as yoghurt, cottage cheese, low-fat or fat-free milk.

Calcium and magnesium help for many of the symptoms associated with menopause, especially headaches, anxiety attacks, hot flushes, insomnia and irritability. They also relieve leg cramps, backache and muscular pain. (Consult chapter 10 on the role of calcium and magnesium.)

6 Other supplements

Other supplements that delay the onset of menopause and alleviate the symptoms include the following:

- Vitamin E and selenium protect against cardiovascular disease by reducing platelet aggregation, which can contribute to heart attacks and stroke. They also alleviate hot flushes and delay the ageing process because of their strong antioxidant action. Use up to 800 IU (664 mg) of vitamin E a day at first and, as the hot flushes improve, reduce the dose to 300-400 IU (249-332 mg).
- Vitamin C (1 000-2 000 mg in divided doses) also alleviates hot flushes.
- Essential fatty acids such as evening primrose oil (1 000 mg a day), linseed oil and salmon oil (500 mg a day) alleviate almost all the symptoms of menopause and prevent the bad LDL-cholesterol levels from increasing. They ensure that the good HDL-cholesterol levels remain high, thereby preventing atherosclerosis (thickening of the arteries).
- Chromium (200 micrograms a day) ensures that the blood sugar levels remain constant, lowers LDL-cholesterol and increases HDL-cholesterol. It also reduces sweet cravings.
- Vitamin A (10 000 IU or 3 030 micrograms or 3 mg of RE activity a day) supports the mucosa and skin. It is a potent antioxidant. Also take beta carotene (25 000 IU or 15 mg a day).
- B-complex vitamins (50 mg of B1-B6, 50 micrograms of B12 and 400 micrograms of folic acid) support the pituitary gland, the nervous system (depression, irritability and tension) and the female urogenital system.
- Iron (15 mg a day) remains important until menstruation stops completely and even for a while afterwards.
- Iodine and kelp (marine algae) are important for supporting the thyroid gland that, in turn, improves female hormone function.
- Zinc (15 mg a day) helps for depression and supports the female urogenital system.

7 Herbal supplements

- Dong quai *(Angelica sinensis)*, or simply angelica, is a popular Chinese herbal remedy that has helped many women. It is non-toxic and is used in Chinese medicine as an anabolic (building up) tonic which improves the blood circulation. Angelica itself does not have any oestrogen or progesterone activity, but it improves the body's own hormone activity. Remember that the female hormones are also produced in the fatty tissue, liver and adrenal glands. Before menopause 50 per cent of the oestrogen is produced in the ovaries and 50 per cent in the other organs. After menopause most of the oestrogen is produced in the other organs and the production of ovarian oestrogen declines markedly. The oestrogen produced by the other organs, known as oestriol, is a much milder and less potent type of oestrogen than the oestradiol produced in the ovaries. Western herbalists and naturopaths often use angelica to treat any disorder of the female urogenital system, such as irregular or painful menstruation (PMS) and menopause. The recommended dose is usually two capsules twice a day or one dropper full of the tincture in a little water twice a day. Angelica is regarded as the most important herbal remedy for keeping the female urogenital system in balance.

- Wild yam *(Dioscorea villosa)* and fenugreek have a progesterone effect to balance the oestrogen effect of unicorn, soya beans and calendula. Wild yam is one of the most commonly used herbs in the world. Unlike synthetic progesterone, natural progesterone does not promote virilisation and fluid retention. It can be applied to the body as a cream (face, abdomen, breasts, back and thighs) once or twice a day for 23 days and then five days' rest or taken in the form of a tea made of the root. It is also available as capsules (about 500 mg a day). The dose can be doubled after two or three months if the symptoms have not cleared up. Progesterone is the most important hormone to supplement during and after menopause. Remember that oestrogen is still made in other organs, but most of the progesterone is made by the ovaries. Natural progesterone from wild yam prevents osteoporosis (some studies claim that it actually reverses osteoporosis). It also helps for vaginal dryness, decreased libido, PMS and painful periods, headache and painful joints.
- The phyto-oestrogens and progesterones in soya beans and other herbs protect against prostate cancer in men and various hormone-dependent diseases such as breast cancer, endometriosis, fibrocystic breast disease (fibroadenosis), painful menstruation (dysmenorrhoea), absence of menstruation (amenorrhoea), uterine myomas and menopausal symptoms in women. Red clover extract has a similar effect. The phyto-oestrogens bind to the same receptors as the

cancer triggering oestrogen and prevent the oestrogen from initiating the cancer process.

I recommend a combination of lifestyle adjustments (stress management and moderate exercise) with supplements (antioxidant combination, calcium and magnesium supplements, essential fatty acids), soya products and herbs such as angelica, chaste tree berry and wild yam. Wild yam works well in the form of a cream or tablets. The dose can be adapted according to bone density evaluation and effective control of symptoms. It can be used quite safely – the right dose is the one that works for you. It can also be used over a long period of time. One source claims up to 90 years – in fact for a lifetime!

- Fennel contains natural plant oestrogen and progesterone. Use it in salads, meat marinades and sauces.
- Sage helps for hot flushes. Make a drink of hot water with honey and three drops of essential oil of sage for night sweats. You can make a tea of fresh sage infused in boiling water for a while. For a good night's rest make a tea of fresh ginger root, sage, camomile, lime blossom and valerian root, with a little honey.
- Ginseng helps to improve energy levels and to reduce fatigue.
- Chaste tree berry *(Vitex agnus castus)* helps to alleviate menopausal symptoms. It increases the production of dopamine, a neurotransmitter in the brain. It prevents breast cancer, reduces breast lumps, alleviates oedema, skin problems, vaginal dryness, hot flushes, period pains and restores mental calm. It clearly has a hormonal effect on the body without any side effects.
- Ginger improves circulation and acts as a gentle stimulant.
- Black cohosh *(Cimicifuga racemosa)*, unicorn root (contains natural oestrogens) and liquorice root are excellent tonics for the female urogenital system. Black cohosh is a well-researched herb that is good for many health problems. The North American Indians use it for bronchitis, whooping cough, asthma, rheumatism, insect bites and snakebite. In the West today it is used mainly for women's health and particularly for menopausal symptoms. It alleviates hot flushes, vaginal dryness and depression. Black cohosh lowers the levels of the luteinising hormone which is secreted by the pituitary gland, the chief cause of hot flushes. Unlike conventional oestrogen replacement therapy, black cohosh does not interfere with the secretion of the other hormones from the pituitary gland. Women can also use it to alleviate menstrual cramps and for arthritis, neuralgia and tinnitus (ringing in the ears). It is best to take it in capsule form

according to the dosages given on the container (usually one capsule twice a day). Black cohosh is a uterine stimulant and should not be taken by pregnant women. It is also contraindicated for women who are breastfeeding because of its oestrogen effect.

● Valerian root helps for anxiety, tension and insomnia.
● St John's wort *(Hypericum perforatum)* and verbena can be used to alleviate emotional problem such as depression. *Ginkgo biloba* is excellent for treating depression, memory loss and cardiovascular disease. Garlic also provides excellent protection against cardiovascular disease.

Always get your herbs from a specialist on herbal therapies. If you have some of the herbs in your garden, use the quantities you would use to flavour food or make a tea. Decide for yourself what suits you best.

Reduce HRT gradually: Do not stop taking your hormone medication too suddenly. Reduce the dose gradually over a period of two or three months while you start using natural products. First halve your dose for ten days, then take the half dose every second day for ten days, then every third day for ten days, etc. The plant progesterones must be taken (or rubbed in) for 23 days and then left for a week so that the receptors remain sensitive to them. If you have already stopped menstruating, this should not start menstruation again as the application and dosage are too low.

Natural plant progesterones improve the effectiveness of the thyroid hormones. Remember to monitor your thyroid medication by having your thyroid stimulating hormones (TSH) levels measured regularly. In due course you may be able to reduce this medication as well.

It takes a while before herbs and supplements start to work (usually two or three months). Give them a fair chance – be patient.

8 Aromatherapy

Aromatherapy oils often help to alleviate the symptoms of menopause. Essential oils of sage, cypress and geranium improve the physical symptoms of menopause. Keep a mixture at hand to inhale when necessary. You could also add six to eight drops to your bath water. For massaging add 15 drops of each of the essential oils to 100 ml of a carrier oil (almond, coconut, olive or grape seed).

Geranium, lavender, grapefruit, camomile, bergamot, neroli, clary sage, vertivert oils and benzoin work well for depression and stress. Add them to your bath water and massage them into the temples, neck or abdomen. Dilute them as described above.

9 Exercise

Exercise is one of the most important and best ways of alleviating symptoms of menopause and stress. Any form of exercise is good for you. The best exercises are those that improve bone density as well. Walking is the best example. Every woman can find the time in her busy daily schedule to do 20 minutes of walking.

Other good exercises include swimming, aerobic exercise, cycling and dancing. Pelvic floor exercises will prevent or retard pelvic muscular degeneration. It is important to do these activities regularly – half an hour five times a week. Exercise also improves symptoms of depression, stress anxiety and the development of atherosclerosis. It ensures a general improvement in health and wellbeing.

10 Smoking

Apart from all the other consequences of smoking, it leads to early symptoms of menopause. Please give up smoking! It also increases the risk of developing osteoporosis and cardiovascular disease.

11 Hormone replacement therapy (HRT)

Hormone replacement therapy (HRT) is a very sensitive subject. Many women are in favour of it, but the number of women who are reluctant to commit themselves is even greater. The pros and cons are briefly presented. Then you can use the information to make an informed choice. You can also decide to try out the natural plant progesterones, oestrogens and other remedies first.

Synthetic oestrogen is prescribed on its own or in combination with progesterone. The combination is prescribed when a woman's uterus is still intact so that the uterine mucosal lining is protected against cancer. Excessive use of oestrogen can cause cancer of the uterus. If a woman's ovaries and uterus have been removed (after a hysterectomy), only oestrogen replacement therapy is prescribed.

Synthetic HRT need not be used indefinitely. It could simply be used for a year or two to overcome the worst symptoms of menopause.

Advantages of hormone replacement therapy

- It prevents osteoporosis.
- It prevents heart attacks and strokes.
- It prevents hot flushes.
- It increases energy levels.
- It improves state of mind and emotional stability.
- It alleviates insomnia.
- It prevents atrophy (thinning) of vaginal mucosal lining.
- It prevents weakening of the pelvic floor muscles.

Disadvantages of hormone replacement therapy

- It increases the chances of developing endometrial cancer (affecting inner lining of the uterus).
- It increases the chances of developing breast cancer.
- It increases the chances of developing thrombosis (blood clots).
- It increases water and salt retention.
- It increases body weight.
- It can cause gall stones.
- It produces PMS symptoms, including tender and painful breasts and fluid retention.
- There is a need for regular medical consultations for checking and follow-up, with cost implications and increased chance for surgical procedures.

Look at all your options and make a choice. A family history of breast or endometrial cancer or venous thrombosis are indications against using HRT. However, if you have a family history of osteoporosis or cardiovascular disease, you could consider HRT. As already stated, you need not use it forever.

Look at the alternatives and decide whether you want to try the natural options and lifestyle changes first. Remember that the natural plant oestrogens and progesterones also provide the same benefits as the synthetic hormone replacements, but with hardly any of the side effects. This is because the whole plant is used in balance and not only isolated active ingredients. The plant progesterones found in wild yam are utilised in the body in other ways. They also act as precursors of oestrogen and the stress hormones (cortisol). Synthetic oestrogen and progesterone are the end products of progesterone synthesis. It is ironic that most of the progestins and progestogens are manufactured from the original wild yam. The active ingredients of the natural plant are isolated in the laboratory and then patented by pharmaceutical companies.

These unopposed end products cause a negative nourishback to the hormone receptors (high synthetic hormone levels send a suppressing message to the other organs that produce oestrogens and progesterones). This means that a woman's body makes less of its own hormones and this can lead to various side effects. Examples are water and salt retention (that increases osteoporosis) and low blood sugar levels. Synthetic progestogens can also aggravate symptoms of PMS and lead to symptoms of virilisation (more hair on the skin, growing a beard, deepening of the voice, etc.), increased risk of breast cancer and high blood pressure. Natural progesterones are actually effective in the treatment of all these symptoms. If you are not satisfied after a few months of natural therapy, you can always decide to change to the conventional HRT.

Remember that low blood sugar is the single most important factor that aggravates hot flushes.

There are many steps you can take to delay the onset of menopausal symptoms, to minimise the menopause and at the same time improve your general health and wellbeing!

19 Micronutrients for the male urogenital system

Throughout the world there is an increased incidence of infertility among men. Sperm counts and motility of sperm are on the decline and the incidence of defective sperm is on the increase. After eliminating physical and hormonal factors, the main causes seem to include high stress levels, poor eating habits, the high production of free radicals in the environment (for example toxins on plants) and in the body, increased hormone levels as a result of hormone additives to food fed to animals, lack of exercise and high alcohol intake. All these lifestyle habits can be changed. Remember that very hot baths, spa baths (jacuzzis) and saunas can reduce sperm production. The same applies to clothing that is too tight.

Other disorders of the male urogenital system are prostate problems, low libido, impotence and chronic fatigue (yuppy flu, fibromyalgia or ME). Many of these problems can be improved with the usual recipe of stress management, healthy eating habits (plenty of fresh fruit and vegetables, wholegrain, as little animal fat as possible), exercise, food supplements and drinking eight glasses of water a day. Remember that increased cholesterol can also cause impotence.

Caffeine and tobacco irritate the prostate. Reduce your intake of sugar, high saturated (animal) fats and refined carbohydrates (white bread and products made from white flour). Beer increases production of prolactin, which indirectly increases the production of dihydro-testosterone, another hormone that causes the prostate cells to multiply. This cell division appears to be the underlying cause of an enlarged prostate.

Benign prostate hypertrophy (BPH), or enlarged prostate, is probably the most common physical complaint in men over the age of 40. It affects 30 per cent of 50 year olds, 50 per cent of 60 year olds and 80 per cent of men above the age of 70. When the prostate enlarges, it constricts the urethra that transports the urine and semen out of the body. BPH thus causes symptoms of changed urination, inability to completely empty the bladder, constant dripping, constant urge to urinate and difficulty in urination. BPH can be a precursor of more serious prostate problems, including damage to and infections of the kidneys and bladder and prostate cancer.

That is why all men over 40 should have an annual prostate examination and a prostate-specific antigen blood test. A balanced diet with plenty of fresh fruit and vegetables and the minimum of saturated animal fat, in addition to rest, relaxation, stress management and exercise are strongly recommended in the treatment of BPH. Improved prostate health can be obtained by voiding the prostate regularly (by ejaculating about three times a week) and daily prostate massage (contracting the pelvic muscles and stopping urine flow, i.e. pinching – ten to 15 muscle contractions a day).

Multivitamin, mineral and antioxidant combination

A few micronutrients that can restore the function to the male urogenital system are discussed. They should contain the usual ingredients already described. Concentrate on the following in particular:

- Vitamin E (400 IU or 332 mg a day) and selenium (200 micrograms a day) are essential for the effective functioning of the reproduction organs in men and women. Vitamin E protects the sex hormones (and other hormones) against oxidation and free radicals. Vitamin E also protects the nucleus in cells from damage by free radicals. The cells of the male urogenital system are very sensitive to a damaged nucleus, which can lead to malfunctions. Active hormone-producing cells have a high oxygen turnover, which produces more free radicals. (Consult Chapter 5 on antioxidants.) Remember that stress, smoking, infections, pollution and overtraining also increase the production of free radicals. Vitamin E has long been regarded as the fertility vitamin; the antioxidants also limit lipid peroxidation which causes a lot of damage by free radicals. By neutralising these, production of hormones and neurotransmitters improves. This in turn improves impotence, fatigue and low libido.

  Selenium reduces the risk of developing prostate cancer. Vitamins E and B6 lower prolactin levels, an important fact in reducing the risk of BPH.
- Vitamin C (1 000 mg a day in divided doses) is an important antioxidant, particularly for smokers and people with longterm high stress levels. Vitamin C is also essential for the synthesis of the male

sex hormones (androgens). In cases of prostatitis (infection of the prostate gland) the recommended dose is 1 000 mg three times a day until the infection clears.

- Zinc (30 mg a day) is probably the most important micronutrient for the normal functioning of the male urogenital system. Semen contains high concentrations of zinc. Zinc supplementation can improve the sperm count and sexual function. Zinc is important in treating infertility, impotence and loss of libido. Pumpkin seeds are an important source of zinc. Pumpkin seeds are also rich in beta-sitosterol, a plant sterol that binds to the testosterone receptors, as well as in vitamin E. Take 60 mg of zinc a day during acute prostatitis and reduce to a maintenance dose of 30 mg a day as soon as the symptoms improve. Long-term stress causes a considerably increased need for zinc. Zinc supplements can reduce copper levels; so it is a good idea to take 1 mg of copper a day with a meal, but not at the same time as the zinc.

- Vitamin A (5 000 IU or 1 515 micrograms or 1,5 mg of RE activity a day) and beta carotene (25 000 IU or 15 mg a day) are important antioxidants for smokers. Vitamin A protects the mucous lining of the genital system against infections and injuries and ensures rapid recovery after infection or injury.

- B-complex vitamins with inositol and choline are important for the normal functioning of the male urogenital system. They improve blood circulation and assist in the maintenance of a normal blood pressure. They also lower cholesterol levels.

Essential fatty acids (omega-3 and omega-6)
Consult Chapter 9. Omega-3 fatty acids found in coldwater fish (salmon, sardines, mackerel) and in specific supplements reduce the risk of BPH.

Calcium, magnesium, et al.
Consult Chapter 10.

Amino acids

- Arginine (2 000-4 000 mg a day on an empty stomach) is recommended for impotence and infertility. Research has shown that it increases the sperm count and the motility of sperm. Arginine stimulates the formation of the male sex hormones. It also stimulates the secretion of the growth hormone in young men and is important for muscular development, muscle power and muscle tone. People with active herpes infection or schizophrenia should not take arginine.

● Taurine (2 000-4 000 mg a day on an empty stomach) can improve the production and motility of sperm.

Medicinal herbs

Consult Chapter 13 on natural alternative to antibiotics for information on herbs that can be used for prostatitis and other infections (herpes, sexually transmitted diseases and bladder infections) of the male urogenital system. Bladder infections in men always warrant further investigation by a medical doctor to eliminate physical causes. Herbs have similar benefits to those of prescription medication, but without the side effects. Herbs act almost imperceptibly and it takes longer to notice the effect. Just be patient.

● Saw palmetto (*Serenoa repens*, 160 mg in a standardised extract twice a day or 30-60 drops in water) is very effective in treating benign prostate hypertrophy (BPH), a very common problem in men over 40. Saw palmetto has a similar effect to that of the expensive pharmaceutical medication finasteride (Proscar): it protects the prostate against the irritating effects of a surplus of testosterone and is more effective. Saw palmetto is non-toxic and can safely be used indefinitely. It prevents the conversion of testosterone into dihydrotestosterone (which stimulates the prostate cells to multiply). Use it with *Pygeum africanum*.

● *Pygeum africanum* (about 100 mg a day) contain phytosterols, especially betasitosterol. Betasitosterol occurs in pumpkin seeds and the recently introduced product containing phytosterols and sterolines isolated from the African wild potato *(Hypoxis rooperi)* and pine nuts. The plant sterols in pygeum (one of which is betasitosterol) strengthens cell membranes and can improve the production of male sex hormones and prostate functioning. It also has an anti-inflammatory effect. The triterpenes in pygeum reduce swelling of the prostate. The ferulic ester bonds reduce prolactin secretion and prevent the accumulation of cholesterol in the prostate. Prolactin increases the prostate's absorption of testosterone. The accumulation of cholesterol increases the number of binding places for the testosterone. (Increased testosterone is the cause of BPH.)

- True ginseng (Asian or Korean, *Panax ginseng*) and the other ginsengs (Siberian and American) are well-known methods for treating prostate problems and increasing libido. They contain ginsenocides that affect and support the hormone activity of the pituitary-adrenal gland axis. Most of the ginsengs (American, Asian and Siberian) increase the body's resistance to stress – they are adaptogens. As such they have the ability to target any system of the body that lacks nutritional support. In this way they improve energy production, metabolism, skin and muscle tone and hormone balance. *Panax ginseng* can increase blood pressure; so if you suffer from hypertension, rather take American ginseng. Make sure that you use a high quality product. It is usually expensive. Ginseng has to be used for a few months before the effects are noticed. You can buy the whole dried root and make a tea of it. Ginseng extract is also available in liquid or capsule form.
- *Ginkgo biloba* (60 mg twice a day) improves peripheral blood flow to the penis and is often successfully prescribed for impotence. Physical, emotional and psychological causes of impotence and erectile dysfunction should always be considered and eliminated first.
- Yohimbe bark has been used for centuries in Africa to treat impotence. Yohimbine extract is prescribed as a medicine and in the United States it is a recognised treatment for impotence. Yohimbine has to be prescribed by a medical doctor. The active ingredient can be toxic to the liver and it can cause a sudden drop in blood pressure.
- Soya products containing plant oestrogens can dramatically reduce the risk of BPH and prostate cancer. All men over the age of 40 should be examined regularly for prostate disorders by a medical doctor.

    Other herbs that are used for balancing the male urogenital system, providing energy and improved stress management include schisandra *(Schisandra chinensis)* and rehmania *(Rehmania glutinosa)*.

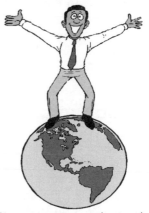

Stress management, exercise, a healthy diet, supplementation and healthy habits will sort out most physical and psychological problems.

20 Natural remedies for the skin

Some of the micronutrients and ingredients that contribute to keeping the skin young and healthy are discussed briefly. The guidelines for a healthy lifestyle also apply, namely healthy eating habits, plenty of water, stress management and exercise. Long-term stress often manifests in skin diseases such as eczema, outbreaks of psoriasis, acne, nettle rash, and skin rashes (dermatitis). Smoking adversely affects the general condition of the skin and accelerates the ageing process.

The skin is the largest organ in the body; it forms a protective layer between ourselves and the outside world. It protects us from environmental toxins, invasion by bacteria, fungi, parasites and viruses and mechanical injury. The skin regulates body temperature, excretes waste matter and is the main organ for the sense of touch. It must be well cared for and looked after.

The factor that contributes most to ageing of the skin – let alone the risk of skin cancer – is sun damage. Everyone should use a sunscreen cream with a protective factor of at least 15 on all parts of the body that are exposed to the sun. Also try to stay out of the sun between 09:30 and 16:00. While a little sun is good for health, try to take your dose of sunlight early in the morning or late in the afternoon, for no longer than 30 minutes a day.

Natural ingredients in sunscreens

Sunscreens all contain cocoa butter (a good moisturiser), para-amino benzoic acid (PABA is a B-complex vitamin that protects the skin from UV-B rays), sesame seed oil (protects against ultraviolet rays, but not enough for a light skin) and zinc oxide (offers complete protection against UV-A and UV-B rays). Research has also shown that supplements of beta carotene and lycopene (the red pigment in tomatoes) reduce sun damage.

Aloe vera contains vitamins, minerals, enzymes and proteins that relieve sunburn and other skin damage, and nourish the skin. Avocado oil and vitamin E nourish and protect the skin. Vitamin C protects the skin from sun damage and increases the levels of vitamin E. Excessive exposure to sun dramatically reduces the skin's vitamin C content. Try to use a sunscreen that contains vitamins C and E. Many researchers claim that covering the skin with a synthetic sunblock can lead to reduced absorption of vitamin D. Vitamin D is important for the prevention of melanoma and basal cell carcinoma. In some cases sunscreens merely delay the sun damage; they do not really prevent it. Vitamin D in a sunscreen absorbs harmful free radicals, improves immunity and controls cell growth, an important factor in preventing skin cancer (such as melanoma and basal cell carcinoma).

Apart from those already mentioned, herbal remedies that help to prevent sun damage and treat irritated skin and bruises include witch hazel *(Hamamelis virginiana)*, milk thistle, cucumber and lavender.

Try a sunscreen and sunblock that contains natural sun protection. Also take a general antioxidant combination with high doses of vitamins A, E and C for internal protection.

Alpha hydroxy fruit acids (AHA)

The alpha hydroxy fruit acids which, as the name suggests, occur in fruit are the only ingredients that have been scientifically proven to delay the ageing process and even to reverse it. This is particularly true of sun damage. AHA stimulates skin renewal and it is particularly good for dry skin. It has been used by dermatologists for more than 30 years for the treatment of adut acne and for age spots. Improvement is usually noticed within two weeks. The fruit acids most commonly used are malic acid (from apples), gluconic acid (from sugar cane), lactic acid and tartaric acid (from red grapes). Marine algae contain pyruvic acid and malic acid with long-chain polysaccharides which make the skin feel soft. Alpha hydroxy fruit acids are also combined with vitamins, minerals and herb extracts.

AHA works through a process of exfoliation of the skin and thus thinning the outer layer (epidermis) of the skin. As a person gets older, the outermost layer of skin thickens, distorting the tissue beneath the skin and forming wrinkles. AHA breaks the connections between the cells of the outer layer of skin and accelerates the sloughing of old, dead cells and stimulates the formation of new cells.

This process can cause skin irritation. Use low-concentration (8-10 per cent), properly buffered (so that the pH is not too low) AHA creams. AHA makes the skin more sensitive to ultraviolet rays. This increases the risk of sun damage and skin cancer. Use AHA at night and apply a natural sunscreen during the day.

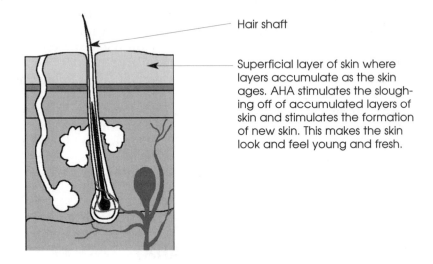

Hair shaft

Superficial layer of skin where layers accumulate as the skin ages. AHA stimulates the slough-ing off of accumulated layers of skin and stimulates the formation of new skin. This makes the skin look and feel young and fresh.

Micronutrient supplementation

The following micronutrient supplements are recommended for a heal-thy skin, all skin complaints and to delay and retard the ageing process:

1 Multivitamin, mineral and antioxidant combination

It is important to neutralise and restrict the potential damage by free radicals that lead to ageing of the skin. (Consult Chapter 5 for more information on antioxidants.) Concentrate on vitamins A, E and C.

2 Essential fatty acids

Essential fatty acids are extremely important for the maintenance of the skin and are used in the treatment of almost all skin complaints. (Consult Chapter 9 for more information.)

3 Calcium, magnesium, et al.

Calcium, magnesium and the rest are essential for strong and healthy hair and nails and for the skin. (Consult Chapter 10 for more information.)

4 Fibres such as bran and psyllium bark

Fibre, taken with plenty of water, prevents the accumulation of toxins in the colon, which can lead to general toxicity in the body, which in turn affects the skin.

5 Amino acids

Amino acids such as L-cysteine, N-acetyl-L-cysteine, methionine and glutamic acid are all important for destroying free radicals and delaying the ageing of skin. (Consult Chapter 5 on antioxidants.) Take 500-1 000 mg of one of the amino acids daily on an empty stomach together with vitamins B6 and C and a little fruit juice to promote cell division, healthy skin and the repair of damaged skin. L-tyrosine, the precursor of the thyroid hormones, is important for the pigmentation of skin and hair. (Consult Chapter 16 on weight management.)

6 Herbs

Herbs can be effectively used for almost all skin complaints:

- Echinacea is excellent for all skin infections, acne and poor lymph drainage. It can be applied to the skin and taken internally. (Consult Chapter 13 on natural alternatives to antibiotics.)
- Golden seal *(Hydrastis canadensis)* can be applied to wounds and taken orally. It helps for infections, insect bites and skin irritations. Research has shown that the berberine in golden seal is very effective for the treatment of psoriasis.
- Comfrey *(Symphytum officinale)* can be made into a paste with baking soda and golden seal and applied to any insect bite or area of skin irritation caused by plants, chemicals or metals and covered with a bandage. It should not be taken internally as that may cause liver damage.

- *Aloe vera* gel is an essential item in any first aid box. It relieves any skin complaint and helps to keep healthy skin in good condition. It can be applied to burns, sunburn and inflamed skin. It also promotes healing of the skin.
- Tea tree oil (*Melaleuca alternifolia,* et al.), from the Australian tea tree plant, is excellent for all skin complaints. It has a strong antiseptic and antifungal effect and can be used for almost all skin infections and skin inflammation such as rosacea. Persistent fungal infections of the nails, hair and skin (athlete's foot, ringworm and candida) respond well to tea tree oil. It relieves eczema, acne, boils, psoriasis, vaginal infections and haemorrhoids (piles) and can also be rubbed on the chest for coughs and colds. Make sure that you buy pure tea tree oil.
- Calendula (*Calendula officinalis*) is a well-known plant that is also a good antiseptic and anti-inflammatory. It is included in various natural preparations for the skin and effective in treating varicose vein ulcers, piles, bruises, mouth ulcers, skin infections, vaginal infections and skin irritations. Apply calendula leaves to a wound to stop bleeding, prevent infection and promote healing. It also improves blood circulation. Add calendula to rice, soup, cheese dishes, yoghurt and omelettes to provide an attractively yellow colour and improve your blood circulation and skin condition.
- Camomile has a healing and calming effect on the skin. It also has anti-inflammatory and antiseptic properties. Camomile promotes healing of wounds and helps for eczema, dermatitis and psoriasis.
- Arnica is a good general remedy for all skin complaints and for keeping a healthy skin in good condition.
- Lavender and origanum (marjoram) – in a combination called thymol – are used to treat aching muscles and to reduce swelling.
- Eucalyptus oil can be rubbed onto aching muscles and joints. It has an antiseptic effect and is good for bacterial and fungal infections of the skin. It helps to clear a blocked nose and congested chest – apply it in the nose and rub it on the chest.

General tips

A good general herbal mixture for the itchy, dry skin associated with acne, eczema and psoriasis should include tea tree oil, witch hazel, *aloe vera*, calendula, golden seal, camomile and arnica. Add Echinacea to this mixture to prevent and treat infections.

A good steam treatment for the face should include rose petals, calendula, camomile and lavender to purify, relax and nourish the skin. Apply moisturiser afterwards.

A good recipe for treating acne is ten drops of tea tree oil, 50 ml rose water, 10 ml fresh witch hazel, 10 ml fresh lavender flowers, 10 ml fresh camomile flowers and 10 ml fresh elder flowers. (If dried flowers are used, take 20 g of each.) Mix the tea tree oil with the rose water and witch hazel to form an astringent. Mix the lavender and the other flowers in a bowl and pour boiling water over them. Steam the face for ten minutes and then apply the astringent. (Consult Chapter 15 for information on acne and teenagers.)

Natural ingredients will set you on the road to recovery for almost any skin complaint and to prevent premature ageing of the skin. Cortisone creams and other potentially harmful ointments are not the only solution to skin problems. Every reader must be convinced by now of the advantages of having one's own herb garden!

21 Micronutrients for the digestive system

The digestive system is responsible for the intake, digestion and absorption of all the nutrients that are needed to nourish every cell in the body, to provide energy for all the biochemical and metabolic processes and to keep the tissues, organs and systems in peak condition.

Remember the saying, 'You are what you eat.' Every single thing you put into your mouth eventually becomes a part of your cells, your emotions and your thought processes. By eating healthy food, managing stress and using supplements, you are ensuring that your body and soul are getting the best possible nutrition.

The mouth, oesophagus, stomach, small intestine, pancreas and colon form the digestive system which is responsible for the digestion and absorption of food. On a more subtle level the emotions, stress levels and hormone balance also affect the process of digestion and absorption.

Most holistic healing disciplines such as Ayurveda and Naturopathy emphasise eating habits and how they affect your general health. In fact, most of the diseases of today can be traced to wrong eating habits.

Receptors for neurotransmitters such as serotonin and for the hormones are also found in the digestive tract. That is why the emotions are so closely linked to the eating process and why so many stress-related diseases manifest in the digestive system. Eating disorders such as anorexia, bulimia and obesity, stomach ulcers, duodenal ulcers, gastritis (inflammation of the mucosa in the stomach), spastic colon (irritable bowel), constipation, chronic diarrhoea and even autoimmune disease such as ulcerative colitis and Crohn's disease come to mind.

Healthy eating habits, stress management, giving up smoking, moderate or no alcohol intake, correct supplementation and exercise will bring relief and in many cases lead to complete recovery for almost all the diseases of the digestive tract.

Micronutrients for optimal well-being

1 Antioxidant and multivitamin combination

Pay particular attention to the following:

- Vitamin A, 5 000-10 000 IU or 1 515-3 030 micrograms or 1,5-3 mg of RE activity a day to protect the mucosa of the digestive tract.
- Beta carotene and other carotenoids, 25 000 IU or 15 mg a day
- Vitamin C, 500 mg twice a day
- Vitamin E, 400 IU or 332 mg a day
- B-complex vitamins

All the other antioxidants will be valuable in reducing the damage caused by toxins and free radicals.

2 Essential fatty acids

Omega-3 and omega-6 fatty acids protect the intestinal mucosa, reduce inflammation and infection and improve the general functioning of the digestive tract. (Consult Chapter 9 on essential fatty acids for quantities.)

3 Amino acids

L-glutamine (500-1 000 mg a day on an empty stomach) is a main component of the connective tissue of the digestive tract. Research has shown that supplementation with glutamine can reduce the permeability of the intestinal wall for toxins, candida and allergens. It should therefore be of value for all disorders of the digestive tract.

4 Medicinal herbs

- Ginger is an excellent herbal remedy for improving digestion. It is a good cure for nausea and motion sickness. Make a tea by simmering fresh ginger root (one teaspoonful finely chopped) in boiling water. Ginger is also included in supplements. Simmer dried ginger, cinnamon and pepper in boiling water and use it with a little honey for almost any kind of digestive problem. It should relieve heart-burn, poor digestion and nausea. Peppermint can have a negative effect on some people (it may aggravate heartburn). Try it to see if it helps for your digestive complaints.

- Camomile is an excellent treatment for an upset stomach, poor digestion, colic and stomach cramps. It can safely be given to babies, children, adults and elderly people. Prepare it as a tea. Let it draw for ten minutes. Ensure that you use a camomile that has a strong aroma; otherwise it will not be effective.
- Bromelain, the enzyme found in pineapple, has an anti-inflammatory effect on the mucosa of the digestive tract (about 100 mg three times a day).

All these herbs can be used for infections of the intestines such as diarrhoea and gastro-enteritis. (Consult Chapter 13 on natural alternatives to antibiotics.)

5 Probiotics and prebiotics

Lactobacillus acidophillus and *Bifidobacterium bifidus* are beneficial bacteria (also known as probiotics) that can be used as supplements to restore the balance of the intestinal flora. This is of particular importance in case of an excessive production of candida after taking antibiotics leading to poor digestion or leaky gut. It is recommended for any disorder of the functioning of the digestive tract. Take two capsules three times a day or eat natural, unflavoured yoghurt with live AB cultures.

Oligosaccharides found in artichokes, asparagus, chicory root, garlic, banana, onion, honey, brown sugar, cereal and barley are known as prebiotics. The body does not absorb oligosaccharides; they act as a source of fibre and bulk in the digestive tract. The beneficial bacteria (probiotics) contain an enzyme that can break down the oligosaccharides (prebiotics) and then use them as food. The bifidobacteria then produce acids that make the colon more acidic thereby putting an end to the growth of harmful bacteria.

Whey is also a prebiotic. Whey is the watery liquid separated from curd when milk has soured. It is available in dried form.

People who add probiotics and prebiotics to their diet may feel a little more bloated, windy and 'crampy' than usual. This shows that the beneficial bacteria are establishing an acidic environment to eliminate the harmful bacteria. The body will adapt in due course and the symptoms will disappear.

Supplements of probiotics and prebiotics offer a safe and effective alternative for dealing with the abnormal functioning of the digestive system. If you consider how important digestion is to general health, supplementation with beneficial bacteria will definitely improve the body's resistance to diseases.

Peptic or duodenal ulcers

This disorder is discussed separately to illustrate the difference that lifestyle habits can make to a common disease.

Long-term stress causes increased acid secretion in genetically susceptible individuals. If the immune system is weakened on account of stress, the bacterium *Helicobacter pylori* takes hold. Continual secretion of acids eventually damages the mucosa of the stomach and an ulcer develops.

H. pylori plays an important role in the development of ulcers and gastritis, which include some of the following symptoms: poor digestion, diarrhoea, stomach ache, bloating and discomfort in the abdomen. By clearing up the infection most of the symptoms of gastritis and ulcers will improve – at least for a while. Most bacteria cannot survive in an acidic environment. However, *H. pylori* produces a chemical reaction which neutralises the acid in the stomach and suppresses the secretion of the digestive enzymes. Then it secretes an enzyme that breaks down the stomach's protective mucosal layer. The fungal infection, Candida albicans, often accompanies *H. pylori* infection. It is even speculated that Helicobacter may play a part in cardiovascular disease, autoimmune disease, psoriasis, allergies, rosacea (a chronic inflammatory skin condition), delayed growth in children and chronic fatigue (ME).

H. pylori can negatively affect the absorption of vitamins, minerals, amino acids and fatty acids. It also exposes the digestive system to parasite infections because it disturbs the balance of the intestinal flora.

Practical alternative hints

The reader should by now be well informed about all the alternative methods of treatment. The following guidelines apply for ulcers, ulcerative colitis, Crohn's disease and almost any other chronic disorder of the gastrointestinal tract:

- Increase the population of beneficial bacteria or flora in the intestine with supplements of *Lactobacillus acidophilus* and *Bifidobacillus bifido* (two capsules three times a day). Eat fresh unflavoured yoghurt. These bacteria create a hostile environment for *H. pylori* and gang (candida, parasites, etc). *L. acidophilus* forms lactic acid and hydrogen peroxide which suppress the growth of *H. pylori*.

  Real ginseng *(Panax schinensis)* promotes the growth of beneficial bacteria.
- Ensure that the mucous lining of your stomach and intestine is healthy so that acid is unable to penetrate and damage it. Vitamin A (5 000-10 000 IU or 1 515-3 030 micrograms or 1,5-3 mg of RE activity a day) and the amino acid L-glutathione (250-500 mg a day on an empty stomach) protect and support the mucosa. They are antioxidants and will counteract the toxins that are secreted by *H. pylori*. A combination of vitamin A, glutathione, vitamin C (500 mg morning and evening) and beta carotene and other carotenoids (20 000 IU or 20 mg a day) will reduce the inflammation of the active *H. pylori* infection and improve the efficiency of the immune system. (Consult Chapter 5 on antioxidants.)
- Essential fatty acids reduce the risk for the development of ulcers. They reduce inflammation and are absorbed by the *H. pylori* where they delay growth. They improve immunity and reduce infection in all digestive tract infections and inflammation.
- Garlic is an effective antibiotic that destroys *H. pylori* and other bacteria. Take the equivalent of two small cloves (about 5 g of garlic) once or twice a day.
- Herbs such as golden seal (hydrastis), berberry *(Berberis vulgaris)* and Oregon grape *(Berberis aquifolium)* contain the active ingredient berberine, a broad spectrum natural antibiotic that is effective against *H. pylori*, other bacteria and overproduction of candida.
- Liquorice root *(Glycyrrhiza alba)* assists in repairing the damaged stomach lining and has been used for decades for treating ulcers and heartburn. It is also an antispasmodic (acts against cramps in the stomach and intestine). Continual use of liquorice root may increase blood pressure. However, if you take liquorice root while the ulcer is active and stop taking it when the ulcer has healed, it should not increase the blood pressure or reduce the potassium

level. There is also a product on the market, deglycyrrhizinated liquorice (DHL) where the glycyrrhizin has been removed. Glycyrrhizin is the ingredient which can cause a potassium deficiency and hypertension.

- Try drinking peppermint tea regularly; it calms the mucosal lining of the whole digestive tract and is excellent for heartburn. However, it does not work for all people. If it doesn't work for you, use camomile tea.

- *Aloe vera* contains antibacterial activity and is a well-known herb for treating stomach ulcers and other digestive problems. Take one teaspoonful after meals.

- Cabbage juice is also an effective cure for ulcers.

- Avoid the following:
  - Coffee (ordinary and decaffeinated), alcohol and tobacco smoke.
  - All products that contain salicylate (such as aspirin) and anti-inflammatories.
  - Milk and dairy products (that may increase acid secretion).
  - Big meals (eat smaller, healthier meals more regularly, every two or three hours).

- Stress management techniques are essential. (Consult Chapters 1 and 2.)

22 Health as an holistic lifestyle adjustment

Ageing is the sum total of all the unrepaired cell and tissue damage that occur during a person's lifetime. Most of the damage is caused by free radicals that are increasingly generated as we get older. Free radicals are formed during all metabolic processes and are also generated by stress, disease, poor nutrition, pollution, smoking, environmental toxins and ultraviolet rays.

Our own antioxidant enzymes cannot cope with this cumulative effect of additional damage. Enzyme activity and availability also decline as we get older. The free radicals damage the cell membrane, the mitochondria (power generators) and also the DNA (nucleus material) in the nucleus of the cell. This hampers cell function and energy production and accelerates the ageing process.

Diseases associated with ageing include cataracts (oxidation of the protein fibres in the lens of the eye), skin damage (oxidation of the epidermis of the skin by ultraviolet rays, dehydration and reduction of collagen), arthritis (wear and tear and oxidation of joints), Alzheimer's disease or dementia (oxidation of the brain tissue), bronchitis and cancer (oxidation of nucleus material) and increased production of free radicals because of smoking, cardiovascular disease and atherosclerosis (oxidation of the blood vessels) and chronic infections (damage caused by free radicals reduces the efficiency of the immune system).

The common denominator in all of these is oxidation caused by the accumulation of free radicals. Add to this a lifetime of negative or suppressed emotions, together with uncontrolled long-term stress, and the whole ageing process is accelerated. The effect of our emotions on every cell in our body cannot be overemphasised. As Solomon said in Proverbs 4:23: 'Guard your heart (i.e. emotions) more than any treasure for it is the source of life.' A positive outlook sends positive messages via the blood and neurotransmitters. Positive messages ensure that the cell functions well and can continue to work well for a long time.

Our bodies are quite capable of reaching a healthy age of 120. Yet few people manage to get to 90. Why is this? The main reason is eating habits, lifestyle, lack of exercise, bottled-up feelings, negative feelings of bitterness, prejudice, resentment and revenge – and too little we do to compensate for and limit the damage by free radicals which are so much part of life in today's world.

Anti-ageing techniques

We can do a lot to delay and retard the ageing process and the diseases associated with old age and eventually reach a ripe, healthy old age. Most people are not afraid of getting older. It is the aches and pains and fear of disability associated with old age that bother us. Another factor is our attitude to life. If you consider that 70 is very old and think that you will probably die at the age of 80 when you're 30, you are programming your mind and body. However, if you enjoy your work and your life and say that you will never retire but work a little less to be able to enjoy your free time, your mind and body will constantly receive messages of joyful exuberance and vitality (joie de vivre). If you are dreading your old age or are not sure what you are going to do when you retire, you will feel that you have lost your sense of purpose in life. Ageing and disease processes then set in at a rapid pace.

All the factors that have already been discussed in the Introduction and first two chapters of this book play an important role in the health of one's body, mind, emotions and spirit as one gets older. Good eating habits and a constant body weight are a sure recipe for gradual ageing. Stress management, relaxation, meditation, prayer, acknowledging negative emotions and, most important, the will and ability to move beyond them are essential techniques to retard and delay ageing. Add a good dose of creative activity and hobbies and your mind and spirit will remain young and motivated. Antioxidant supplements help the body to limit the damage by free radicals and thereby ensure that systems function efficiently. Regular cleansing of the mind, body, emotions and soul will help the ageing process to occur gently and gradually. The process of getting old then becomes a rich, joyous experience, full of graciousness, serenity, wisdom and dignity, with a fit and active body and a clear mind – something to look forward to.

Try the following suggestions and see if you feel any younger, more energetic and full of life:

Ten-point plan for gentle cleansing and detoxification

We have all experienced the need and desire to cleanse and purify our bodies and rid ourselves of accumulated waste. This instinct is as old as humankind itself. Throughout history people have undergone various cleansing rituals to purify their minds and bodies of negative emotions and physical waste.

Hot baths, steam baths and periods of fasting help to rid the body of toxins. In addition, herbs, food supplements and a wholesome diet will help to complete and maintain the process of detoxification.

1 Drink water and a herbal mixture

Drink at least eight glasses of water and at least three cups of a cleansing herbal mixture every day. Make an infusion of one teaspoon of dried herbs or two teaspoons of fresh herbs in boiling water and drink it as a tea. Use any of the following herbs on their own or in combination: dandelion, fennel, rosemary, cinnamon, ginger, turmeric or milk thistle. Herbs support the liver, lymphatic system, urinary tract, skin and intestinal canal to get rid of toxins. Add a teaspoon of honey if you like.

2 Balanced diet

Follow a healthy wholesome and balanced diet. Remember the fresh fruit and vegetables, wholegrain products, beans, seeds, pulses and nuts (organically grown if possible). Use garlic, onion, ginger and some of the herbs listed above to prepare tasty and healthy food. Eat plenty of broccoli, cabbage, dark leafy greens, tomatoes and pawpaws. Avoid preservatives, pesticides and chemicals in foods as far as possible. Use monounsaturated fats and unsaturated fats such as olive oil, grape seed oil, flax or linseed oil and canola oil moderately in food preparation and salad dressings. Avoid fried foods, white sugar, white flour, saturated and trans fatty acids (such as animal fats and block margarine). Restrict your intake of caffeine and alcohol and avoid unnecessary medication as far as possible.

3 Fasting

Try to fast for one day a week. A Monday is usually a good idea, but any day will do. Drink at least 12 glasses of water and fruit juices such as apple or grape juice. If you get very hungry, eat an apple or a bunch of grapes. Fasting once a week does wonders for your health and state of mind – and to delay the ageing process. People who suffer from diabetes, other serious diseases and pregnant women should consult their doctors before fasting. Most people can afford to give their digestive tract and metabolism a break one day a week.

4 Exercise

Try to exercise for 20 minutes every day or for 20-30 minutes three or four times a week. It is not necessary to exhaust yourself. A quick walk outdoors, doing dance routines on the lounge carpet or a few lengths in the swimming pool are quite enough. Choose an activity that you enjoy. Finish your exercise session with relaxation exercises. Yoga refreshes your body, give you energy and strength and calm your mind and soul.

5 Steam baths/saunas

Treat yourself to a steam bath once a week. Put five cups of Epsom salts in bathwater as hot as you can stand or have a sauna at the gym. Drink plenty of water or herbal tea while you sweat out your toxins.

6 Micronutrients

Take your micronutrients every day: an antioxidant, multivitamin and mineral combination with calcium, magnesium, et al. and your essential fatty acids. Pay particular attention to vitamin E, B-complex vitamins, co-enzyme Q10, zinc, vitamin C and *Ginkgo biloba*. Add to this an antioxidant amino acid to assist in fat combustion (such as L-glutamine, L-carnitine, choline, L-methionine or L-glutathione). Choose the medicinal herbs and supplements that will best serve your specific needs by supplementing for the system where you have a problem.

7 Fibre

Increase your intake of roughage by sprinkling psyllium seeds, linseeds or bran over your porridge or adding them to salads or food every day. Eat oatmeal porridge. If you take psyllium seeds or linseeds on their own, drink at least one glass of water as well.

8 Beneficial bacteria

Increase the population of 'friendly' bacteria in your intestines by eating fresh, unflavoured yoghurt every day. Otherwise you can take *Lactobacillus acidophilus* or *Bifidobacterium bifidus* capsules – two capsules three times a day.

9 Lust for life

Laugh every day. Solomon also said, 'Gladness of heart gives us life; joy gives us longevity.' It is your choice. Humour supports the immune system, endocrine system and nervous system. The message of positivity and enthusiasm goes to every cell in the body and strengthens your entire being.

10 Gratefulness

Say thank you for at least five good things in your life every day. Do your daily relaxation exercises, including meditation, prayer and quiet time. This calms the mind and nourishes the body. By focussing on the riches we receive every day of our lives we move beyond the wrongs, the negatives, shortcomings and other little things we often choose to focus on.

The most important thing in all our lives is to realise that there must be a balance between body, soul, emotions and intellect. It is not the things you do now and then that make a difference, but the things you do every day of your life as part of your lifestyle.

References

Books

1. 1996. *Natural Medicine – Reader's Digest South African Family Guide.* Reader's Digest Association, South Africa.
2. 1996. *Vitamins in Nutrition and Health.* Vitamin Information Centre.
3. Altenberg, Henry Edward (M.D.). 1992. *Holistic Medicine: A Meeting of East and West.* Japan Publications.
4. Bender, D.A. 1992. *Nutritional Biochemistry of the Vitamins.* Cambridge University Press.
5. Bendich, A. et al. 1990. *Micronutrients and Immune Functions.* New York Academy of Sciences.
6. Bendich, Gaby et al. 1991. *Vitamin Intake and Health.* Marcel Dekker.
7. Benson, Dr Herbert (M.D.). 1996. *Timeless Healing: The Power and Biology of Belief.* Simon and Schuster.
8. Buist, Dr Robert. 1995. *The Cholesterol Myth.* Struik Publications.
9. Chopra, Dr Deepak (M.D.). 1994. *Perfect Weight.* Quantum Publishers.
10. Chopra, Dr Deepak (M.D.). 1993. *Ageless Body, Timeless Mind.* Random House.
11. Drury, Nevill (ed.) 1985. *Inner Health.* Prism Press.
12. Dyer, Wayne (Ph.D. Psych.). 1989. *You'll See It When You Believe It.* HarperCollins.
13. Dyer, Wayne (Ph.D. Psych.). 1992. *Real Magic.* HarperCollins.
14. Dyer, Wayne (Ph.D. Psych.). 1995. *Your Sacred Self.* HarperCollins.
15. Ganong, W.F. 1987. *Review of Medical Physiology.* Appleton & Lange.
16. Giller, Robert M. (M.D.). 1994 *Natural Prescriptions.* Ballantine Books.
17. Goleman, Daniel (Ph.D.). 1996. *The Meditative Mind.* J.P. Tarcher.
18. Grieve, M. (F.R.H.S.). 1994. *A Modern Herbal.* Jonathan Cape Ltd.
19. Haas, Elson M. (M.D.). 1992. *Staying Healthy with Nutrition.*

Celestial Arts Publishers.
20. Hall, Doriel. 1996. *Healing with Meditation.* Gill & Macmillan.
21. Hoad, Judith. 1996. *Healing with Herbs.* Gill & Macmillan.
22. Jacobs, Maryce M. 1991. *Vitamins and Minerals in the Prevention and Treatment of Cancer.* CRC Press.
23. Kenton, Leslie. 1995. *Passage to Power:* Natural Menopause Revolution. Hay House.
24. Lee, John R. (M.D.). 1993. *Natural Progesterone: The Multiple Roles of a Remarkable Hormone.* BLL Publishing.
25. Machlin, Lawrence J. (ed.) 1984. *Handbook of Vitamins: Nutritional, Biochemical and Clinical Aspects.* New York Academy of Sciences.
26. Marti, James E. 1998. *The Alternative Health & Medicine Encyclopaedia.* Visible Ink Press.
27. Meyer, B.J. 1988. *Die Fisiologiese Basis van Geneeskunde.* HAUM Publishers.
28. Michal, Mina. 1991. *Stress: Signs, Sources, Symptoms, Solutions.* Editiones Roche.
29. Mindell, Dr Earl. 1994. *The Herb Bible.* Random House.
30. Mindell, Dr Earl. 1994. *The Vitamin Bible.* Arlington Books.
31. Myss, Caroline (Ph.D.). 1997. *Anatomy of the Spirit.* Bantam Books.
32. Ody, Penelope. 1995. *Home Herbal.* Dorling Kindersley.
33. Passwater, Richard A. (Ph.D.). 1978. *Cancer Prevention and Nutritional Therapies.* Keats Publishers.
34. Polunin, M. & Robbins, C. 1992. *The Natural Pharmacy.* Dorling Kindersley.
35. Prasad, Kedar N. (Ph.D.). 1994. *Vitamins in Cancer Prevention and Treatment.* Healing Arts Press.
36. Roberts, Margaret, 1994. *A-Z of Herbs.* Southern Book Publishers.
37. Rodwell Williams, Sue. 1994. *Basic Nutrition and Diet Therapy.* Mosby.
38. Selye, H. 1976. *Stress in Health and Disease.* Butterworths.
39. Shealy, Norman (M.D.) & Myss, Caroline (Ph.D.) 1993. *The Creation of Health.* Stilpoint Publishing.
40. Shils, Olson & Shike. 1993. *Modern Nutrition in Health and Disease* (Volumes 1 & 2). Lea and Febiger.
41. Siegel, Dr Bernie (M.D.). 1991. *Peace, Love and Healing: The Path to Self-healing.* HarperCollins.
42. Siegel, Dr Bernie (M.D.). 1993. *Living, Loving and Healing: A*

Guide to a Fuller Life, More Love and Greater Health. HarperCollins.

43. Van der Merwe, Dr Arien (M.D.). 1997. *To Health! Health, Stress & Lifestyle Management.* CC Publishers.

44. Van Wyk, Prof. Ben-Erik et al. 1997. *Medicinal Plants of South Africa.* Briza Publications.

45. Wardlaw, G.M. & Insel, P.M. 1996. *Perspectives in Nutrition.* Mosby.

46. Weil, Andrew (M.D.). 1991. *Spontaneous Healing.* Little, Brown & Company (UK).

47. Weil, Andrew (M.D.). 1997. *Natural Health, Natural Medicine.* Warner Books.

48. Werbach, M.R. (M.D.) & Murray, M.T. (N.D.). 1994. *Botanical Influences on Illness: A Sourcebook of Clinical Research.* Third Line Press.

Research papers – A short selection of recent and past research

1. Anderson, R.A. et al. Supplemental chromium effects on glucose, insulin, glucagon and urinary chromium losses in subjects consuming controlled low-chromium diets, *The American Journal of Clinical Nutrition* 1991, No 54: pp. 909-916.
2. *Antioxidant Vitamin Newsletter,* 1992-1998, Nos 1-17.
3. Bender, D.A. B Vitamins in the nervous system, *Neurochem. Int.* 1984, Vol. 6, No 3: pp. 297-321.
4. Benton D. et al. Vitamin supplementation for 1 year improves mood, *Neuropsychobiology* 1995, No 32: pp. 98-105.
5. Benton, D. et al. The impact of long-term vitamin supplementation on cognitive functioning, *Psychopharmacology* 1995, No 117: pp. 298-305.
6. Benton, D. Symposium on nutrition and cognitive efficiency, *Proceedings of the Nutrition Society* 1992, No 51: pp. 295-302.
7. Berdanier, Carolyn D. The many faces of stress, Ph.D., *Nutrition Today,* March/April 1987: pp. 12-17.
8. Briggs, Stephanie. Magnesium: A forgotten mineral, Ph.D., *Health & Nutrition Breakthroughs,* November 1997.
9. Burtis, W.J. et al. Dietary hypercalciuria in patients with calcium oxalate kidney stones, *The American Journal of Clinical Nutrition* 1994, No 60: pp. 424-429.
10. Cohen & Williamson, Stress and infective disease in humans, *Psychological Bulletin* 1991, Vol. 109, No 1: pp. 5-24.
11. Connor et al. Essential fatty acids: The importance of N-3 fatty acids in the retina and brain, *Nutrition Reviews,* Vol. 50, No 4: pp. 21-29.
12. Coutsoudis, A. et al. Vitamin A supplementation reduces measles morbidity in young African children: A randomized, placebo-controlled, double-blind trial, *The American Journal of Clinical Nutrition* 1991, No 54: pp. 890-895.
13. DHA and Neurological/Visual Disorders, *Scientific Abstracts Advanced Medical Nutrition,* May 1998.
14. Goode et al. Changing the nation's diet: A study of responses to correct nutritional messages, *Health Education Journal* 1996, No

55: pp. 285-299.

15. *Health & Nutrition Breakthroughs and Nutrition Science News,* website http://www.nutritionsciencenews.com

16. *Health & Nutrition Breakthroughs,* All publications 1996-1998.

17. Hunt et al. Metabolic responses of menopausal women to supplemental dietary boron and aluminum during normal and low magnesium intake: Boron, calcium and magnesium absorption and retention and blood mineral concentrations, *The American Journal of Clinical Nutrition* 1997, No 65: pp. 803-813.

18. Hussey, G.D. et al. A randomized, controlled trial of vitamin A in children with severe measles, *New England Journal of Medicine,* 19 July 1990, Vol. 323, No. 3: pp. 160-164.

19. Labadarios et al. Blood vitamin concentrations during the acutephase response, *Critical Care Medicine,* Vol. 20, No 7.

20. Labadarios, Weich et al. Plasma vitamin A, E, C and B6 levels in myocardial infarction, *SAMJ,* 2 May 1987, Vol. 71.

21. Le Bars, P.L. et al. A placebo-controlled, double-blind, randomized trial of using an extract of ginkgo biloba for Alzheimer's dementia, *Journal of the American Medical Association,* 22 October 1997, No 278: pp. 1327-1332.

22. Long-term effects of calcium supplements on bone loss and fractures in postmenopausal women: A randomized controlled trial, *American Medical Journal* 1995, No 98: pp. 331-335.

23. Look et al. Serum selenium, plasma glutathione and erythrocyte glutathione peroxidation levels in asymptomatic versus symptomatic human immunodeficiency virus (HIV-1) infection, *European Journal of Clinical Nutrition* 1997, No 51: pp. 266-272.

24. Losonczy, K.G. et al. The use of vitamin C and E and the risk of all-cause and coronary heart disease mortality in older persons, *The American Journal of Clinical Nutrition* 1996, No 64: pp. 190-196.

25. Marine oils and their effects, *Drevon Nutrition Reviews,* Vol. 50, No 4: pp. 38-45.

26. Markus et al. Influence of lifestyle modification on atherosclerotic progression determined by ultrasound change in common carotid intima-media thickness, *The American Journal of Clinical Nutrition* 1997, No 65: pp. 1000-1004.

27. Medical Update *Vitamin Information Centre Nl,* April 1990 - December 1997, Nos. 1-27.

28. Ness et al. Vitamin C status and respiratory function, *European Journal of Clinical Nutrition* 1996, No 50: pp. 573-579.

29. *Nutrition Science News,* All publications 1996-1998.

30. Nygard, Ottar et al. Plasma homocysteine levels and mortality in patients with coronary artery disease, *The New England Journal of Medicine*, 24 July 1997, Vol. 337, No 4: pp 230-236.

31. Orenstein, Neil S. Essential fats help relieve diabetes and osteoporosis, Ph.D., *Health News Naturally*, Keats Publishing, May 1998.

32. Pellegrini, N. et al. Composition of platelet phospholipids after moderate consumption of red wine in healthy volunteers, *European Journal of Clinical Nutrition* 1996, No 50: pp. 535-541.

33. Peters et al. Vitamin C supplementation reduces the incidence of post-race symptoms of upper respiratory tract infection in ultramarathon runners, *The American Journal of Clinical Nutrition* 1993, No 57: pp. 170-174.

34. Psychological stress and susceptibility to the common cold, The *New England Journal of Medicine*, 29 August 1991, Vol. 325, No 9.

35. Psychoneuroendocrinology of stress and its immune consequences, *Antimicrobial Agents and Chemotherapy*, January 1994: pp. 1-6.

36. Psychoneuroimmunology: The interface between behavior, brain & immunity, *American Psychologist*, December 1994: pp. 1004-1017.

37. Santosh-Kumar et al. Unpredictable intra-individual variations in serum homocysteine levels on folic acid supplementation, European Journal of Clinical Nutrition 1997, No 5: pp. 188-192.

38. Schaafsma G. Bioavailability of calcium and magnesium, *European Journal of Clinical Nutrition* 1997, No 51: pp. S13-S16

39. Stephenson et al. Vitamin A is excreted in the urine during acute infection, *The American Journal of Clinical Nutrition* 1994, No 60: pp. 388-392.

40. *Stress and Cancer Psychological Bulletin* 1981, Vol. 89, No 3: pp. 369-406.

41. The activated neutrophil: Formidable forces unleashed, *SAMJ*, October 1995, Vol. 85, No 10.

42. The impact of infection on vitamin metabolism: An unexplored area, *The American Journal of Clinical Nutrition*, September 1977, No 30: pp. 1473-1477.

43. The role of antioxidant vitamins, *The American Journal of Medicine Health Promotion and Disease Prevention*, 26 September 1994, Vol. 2.

44. Thomas, M.K. et al. Hypovitaminosis D in medical inpatients, *New England Journal of Medicine*, 19 March 1998, Vol. 338, No 12: pp. 777-783.

45. Van Elswyk, Mary E. Omega-6 and Omega-3: Essential fatty acids, Ph.D., College of Agriculture and Life Sciences, Texas AM University.

Index

Further information

Dr. Arien van der Merwe is a medical doctor with extensive experience in natural medicine. She is a stress management consultant, a corporate wellness programmer and acts as wellness advisor to various magazines, websites and corporations.

Regular presentations of Dr van der Merwe's published works are presented countrywide. These include lectures, programmes, talks, lunchhour, one-day and weekend workshops, seminars and wellness walks.

Subjects covered include the following:
- Health and wellbeing
- Stress management: Free yourself from fear and worry
- Dynamic corporate wellness and executive health
- Increasing productivity, activity and quality of life
- High cholestorol, high blood pressure, high stress – What Now?
- Reducing absenteeism, promoting personal power, enhancing energy, improving immunity and achieving longevity
- Health risk assessments including all levels of wellbeing
- Mind, body, emotions and soul integration

Programmes can also be custom designed and CD's, video and audio cassette tapes are available.

Further information can be obtained from:
Health, Stress & Lifestyle Management
Cell +27-83-731-2049 or e-mail arienvdm@samedical.co.za